Edward Smith

Consumption

Its Early and Remediable Stages

Edward Smith

Consumption
Its Early and Remediable Stages

ISBN/EAN: 9783743640832

Printed in Europe, USA, Canada, Australia, Japan

Cover: Foto ©Suzi / pixelio.de

More available books at **www.hansebooks.com**

CONSUMPTION:

ITS EARLY AND REMEDIABLE STAGES.

BY

EDWARD SMITH, M.D., LL.B., F.R.S.,

ASSISTANT PHYSICIAN TO THE HOSPITAL OF CONSUMPTION AND DISEASES OF THE CHEST, BROMPTON;
PHYSICIAN TO THE ROYAL DRAMATIC COLLEGE; CORRESPONDING MEMBER OF THE
ACADÉMIE DES SCIENCES, MONTPELLIER, AND OF THE NATURAL
HISTORY SOCIETY OF MONTREAL.

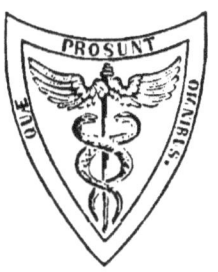

PHILADELPHIA:

BLANCHARD AND LEA.

1865.

DEAR SIR JAMES,

On considering the Medical History of Consumption in our own time, it is impossible not to perceive in how great a degree the profession has been indebted to you for the enlightened views in reference to the early or predisposing conditions of Phthisis, which were propounded in your work published in 1835. But the obscurity which has long rested upon the disease has deterred from, rather than invited to, scientific investigation; and hence, whilst the disease is still as fatal as it was many years ago, and the necessity for a new line of practice universally admitted, there has not been that general attention to the remediable period which the importance of the subject has merited.

It is with the view of again challenging professional inquiry in a direction somewhat similar to that which you pointed out, that the following work has been written; and, although the views to be advanced may not altogether accord with your own, I trust that they may meet with your general approval.

To no one could a work on the early or remediable stages of Phthisis be so fitly inscribed, and I am gratified that you have done me the honour to accept this small tribute of my deep respect and esteem.

I have the honour to be,

Dear Sir James,

Your most sincere and grateful servant,

EDWARD SMITH.

PREFACE.

THE author, in writing the following work, has had four principal objects in view, viz., to take advantage of the growing belief of the day, that there is a stage of Phthisis in which the disease is as remediable as it is irremediable at a later period; to write a practical work in which may be faithfully represented the actual condition of these cases when regarded in the great numbers in which they have been brought before his observation; to treat the subject, as far as possible, on the inductive method, and on the improved physiology and pathology of the day; and to give practical effect to numerous series of special inquiries which have been made by him during the preceding seven years.

It is not important, in reference to the first, that the views differ as to the limits, characteristics, and designation of the early stage, since, when the existence of the stage shall have been well established, an agreement as to its nature will certainly follow. Numerous authorities from distant ages, both as to Phthisis in general and the early stage in particular, are cited; and whilst the author has not omitted to state his own views, he has generally founded his observations rather upon the agreements than the disagreements of individual observers.

In seeking to make the work practical the author has entered largely into all the questions which relate to food, exertion, climate, and others constituting hygienics, because such is in accordance with general feeling at the present time; because this part of medical knowledge is now being placed upon the sure footing of scientific research; and because it must be through the conditions of the everyday life of the patient that medicinal and other remedial agents may influence the constitution in so chronic a disease. For the same reason minute details have been considered of great importance, since it is upon them that the efficient working of a general plan will essentially depend.

The arrangement of the work upon physiological and pathological indications and the use of propositions will, it is hoped, conduce to clearness of exposition and facility of reference, whilst it may also dissociate the consideration of the treatment from that of the evidences, and cause the same conditions or remedies to be viewed under various aspects. It cannot be doubted that assigning views as to the reasons for any particular course will be welcomed by an intelligent and inquiring Profession, whether universally or only partially allowed to be just; and also that it may tend to promote inquiry in thoughtful minds; but in order to summarize the whole plan of treatment the various recommendations have been collected together in one chapter and given in an empirical manner. In reference to the author's special investigations, which have been embodied in the work, it is only necessary to ask attention to the explanation offered at the end of the work, in reference to a statistical inquiry of great extent, which was completed whilst the sheets were passing through the press.

London: 16, Queen Anne Street, W.,
April, 1862.

TABLE OF CONTENTS.

CHAPTER III.

HISTORICAL SKETCH AS TO THE VIEWS IN THE EARLY STAGE OF PHTHISIS.

PART II.

NATURE AND EVIDENCES OF THE EARLY STAGE OF PHTHISIS.

CHAPTER IV.

GENERAL OBSERVATIONS.

CHAPTER V.

CHAPTER VI.

ALIMENTATION.

CHAPTER VII.

ELIMINATION.

CHAPTER VIII.

CHAPTER IX.

CHAPTER X.

CHAPTER XI.

CHAPTER XXI.

THE LUNGS.—EXTERNAL PULMONARY EVIDENCES OF PHTHISIS.

CHAPTER XXII.

THE LUNGS.—INTERNAL PULMONARY EVIDENCES OF EARLY PHTHISIS.

CHAPTER XXIII.

PATHOLOGY OF THE FIRST STAGE OF PHTHISIS AND TUBERCLE.

PART III.

TREATMENT.

CHAPTER XXV.

RESTORE THE BULK OF THE BODY BY LESSENING ELIMINATION.

CHAPTER XXVI.

RESTORE THE BULK OF THE BODY BY LESSENING ELIMINATION.

CHAPTER XXVII.

RESTORE THE BULK OF THE BODY BY INCREASING THE SUPPLY.

CHAPTER XXVIII.

INCREASE THE VITAL ACTIONS.

CHAPTER XXIX.

INCREASE THE ASSIMILATION OF FOOD.

— ...

PART IV.

PROGNOSIS.

CHAPTER XLIV.

CHAPTER XLV.

PROGNOSIS.

CONSUMPTION.

PART I.

INTRODUCTORY AND HISTORICAL.

CHAPTER I.

PRELIMINARY OBSERVATIONS.

THE word consumption almost universally suggests an incurable condition, and one which proceeds slowly yet steadily to its termination, so that there is without doubt in the public mind a greater dread of it than of any other chronic disease. This is well based upon the facts of the widely spread cases of the disease, the opportunity which nearly all persons have of tracing its progress from a certain point, and the multitudes who die from it; but on reflection it will be seen that all this may be true, and yet the inference which has been drawn may be unsound, for it only proves that consumption is not commonly cured, and not that it is incurable. Indeed, admitting as we do the general truthfulness of the received opinions, we feel assured that there are good grounds for believing both the apparently contradictory statements, viz., that consumption is commonly fatal, and yet is commonly curable; and we do this without assuming that there has been any want of due investigation as to the nature, or of care and talent in the treatment of the disease.

In reference to the nature of the disease in past ages, we think that there are some reasons for believing that it was not precisely the same then as now, as, for example, in the inflammatory tendency which was common in the seventeenth, eighteenth, and the early part of the nineteenth century, and which is rare now; and hence, we shall not be justified in adducing former experience, either in aid of, or in opposition to, the present opinion. But the most widely spread source of fallacy is the fact that neither the profession nor the public has taken cognizance of the disease in its early manifestation, but has admitted its existence only after much advance has been made, and then watching the case from that starting-point,

2

it has been seen that the disease is almost universally fatal. If that starting-point were the earliest period at which we could become acquainted with the disease, then we think that the popular belief could not be gainsaid. Hence, the whole question turns upon that point, viz., the general recognition both by the profession and the public of the disease in its earliest manifestations.

In this view it is easy to admit that the present age might be right in believing consumption to be curable, whilst former ages were equally right in their confirmed belief of the contrary : for, until our improved means of diagnosis were discovered and widely known, and cases of the disease were brought together in large numbers for careful investigation and study, it was quite impossible either for the public or the mass of medical practitioners, to do otherwise than commence their recognition of the disease at an advanced period in its progress. Then the disease seemed involved in mystery as to its nature, and so hopeless was it in its progress that practically little attempt was made to control it ; but, at present, we have means of tracing conditions pre-existent to those which constituted the starting-point of former times ; and, notwithstanding the disputation which still exists as to the nature of the material deposited in the lungs, which is said to be the essence of the disease, we venture to affirm that but few diseases are more clear in their nature, or more readily capable of detection in their early manifestations. It is common to speak of the mysterious character of phthisis, as though we assumed that there were other conditions of disease which were more clear, forgetting that we are unacquainted with the essential processes by which either healthy or unhealthy nutrition is carried on, and with the nature of the various conditions of disease to which we have given names. In all these instances we are acquainted with certain leading facts, whilst the minute changes which they grossly represent are hid from view ; and in like manner, and in various degrees, we possess certain powers by which we may violently arrest the processes upon which the diseased action appears to depend ; but in all, our duty is chiefly confined to aiding the efforts of nature. In truth we doubt, with so high an authority as Sir James Clark, if the want of success which has attended our efforts to arrest the progress of phthisis is greater than has attended all efforts to arrest the progress of any other disease, accompanied by an equal destruction of the organ with which it is associated ; and it is only the great prevalence of the disease, and the vast importance of the organ affected in relation to the animal economy, which has led to the present belief of the special incurability of phthisis. It need not be affirmed that we are equally powerless to restore the structure or the function of the liver, or of any other organ on which an equal amount of injury has been inflicted.

Hence, we infer that whilst the present belief may be true under existing conditions, the opprobrium which has specially been cast upon the healing art in reference to phthisis, is at least in great part undeserved; and that now, admitting the practical incurability of the disease after it has made a certain degree of progress, it is our duty to look at the disease in its earlier aspect, and in doing so, to lay aside opinions founded upon facts belonging to a later stage, so that with unprejudiced minds we may ascertain if in that new condition we have not the materials by which the remedial art may act more effectually, and a disease which is in its nature curable.

There is one leading particular in reference to this question in which the present is less unprejudiced than former ages. From the days of Hippocrates to those of Laennec, the disease was distinguished by its general symptoms almost exclusively; but Laennec introduced a new era, in which the state of the lungs took precedence of that of the general symptoms, and tubercle came to be regarded as the essence, the mark, and the starting-point of the disease. This view was a tangible one, because the tubercle was to be seen by every observer; and by the proposition, only tuberculous cases were regarded as phthisical, so that it was generally adopted, and has necessarily influenced the opinions of men educated in it, and who, from its recent occurrence, have lately lived, or are still living. Those who have been more recently educated, or who will hereafter enter upon the study of the subject, will probably regard this question with greater breadth and fairness.

In considering this question, it must be remarked that the tubercle is not the cause, but only one consequence of the disease. This, at the present moment, is in part practically admitted, and in other part as practically denied. It is admitted, inasmuch as there has been an attempt to assign it an origin either in the place where it is found or in the general depraved circulation; and even to this hour the latter source is constantly referred to. But, on the other hand, the changes which occur in the deposited tubercle have been carefully watched, and the progress of destruction of the lung, with all its consequences, has been attributed to the changes which take place in the tubercle, and the tubercle has become the foundation of the disease. It must be admitted that the tubercle is almost universally regarded as the essential feature of the disease, the cause of its progress in the lungs, and the source of injury to the general system; and the great desideratum has been its removal. The general system has been regarded in two aspects: as associated with the deposition of tubercle, and as influenced by the deposition; and the evil has not been in regarding it in this double light, but in giving an undue prominence to the latter, when considering the relation of tubercle to phthisis. In truth, modern views have so engrossed the mind, that one condition in the progress of phthisis has (because it is always found at some period) been raised from the minor to the dignity of the major premiss; and instead of the statement that all cases of tubercle (in the lungs) are phthisis, it is averred that in all cases of phthisis there is tubercle.

We venture to affirm that this consideration is worthy of careful attention in any attempt to obtain a true view of the nature of this disease.

If tubercle be due to pre-existent causes, whatever may be their nature, the disease is not in the tubercle, but in the cause of the tubercle; and the tubercle itself is but a result—an evidence, and all the changes in the tubercle are secondary influences. It cannot be affirmed that the tubercular element of the disease possesses an innate power of destruction such as is found in the elements of cancer, for whatever may be the origin of tubercle in the lung, it is found upon free surfaces, and does not spread by extension; whilst cancer infiltrates the tissues and has the power of extension, and consequently of displacement or destruction. Tubercle itself is a foreign but a passive agent; and all actions, of whatever kind, which proceed about it, originate and are carried on, not by the tubercle, but by the containing tissues. It is placed in the lungs, and accumulates by new deposits; and the subsequent changes are not due to any disintegrating action in the tubercular element, but in the tissues which contain it.

Hence surely the tubercle is not the essence of the disease, but only one of the results—a result doubtless met with at some, but not at every period in the progress of each case. So long as inquirers fix their attention upon this or any other single product of the disease, they will fail to recognize its true nature; and so long as the aim of the practical man is to find a plan whereby the tubercle may be absorbed or ejected, he also will fail. We therefore think that whilst our age has made the great advance of distinguishing more carefully those cases of wasting which are associated with a particular disease of the lungs from those due to other causes, and has therefore given to us a large group of cases of a similar character, it has greatly erred in fixing its attention upon one of the conditions of the lungs, and regarding it, not as one of many results of diseased action, but as the essence of the disease, and the prime cause of mischief. It has cast aside that minute attention to the general system which was the especial subject of observation of the fathers of medicine, and has been content to concentrate all its powers of observation upon one internal condition which has this in common with the external symptoms, viz., that both are effects of the disease, and not the disease itself. We have limited our cases to one class only, and have spent our time in determining the characteristics of that class, but have made little progress in that higher department of knowledge—the determination of the true nature of the disease.

CHAPTER II.

HISTORICAL SKETCH AS TO THE NATURE AND TREATMENT OF PHTHISIS.

WE do not purpose in the following sketch of the opinions which have been hitherto held respecting phthisis, to enter into large detail, but we desire rather to trace the changes of opinion or the additions to the knowledge of the disease which have occurred in large eras of medical history, with a view to show the real amount of progress which has been made since the days of the earliest records of our art. This may be in part effected by the aid of the labours of Dr. Young, to whom the profession is indebted for abstracts of the works of nearly all preceding writers on consumption—accurate, no doubt, and arranged in chronological order, but having the great defect of an absence of scientific arrangement in the direction of the present inquiry, and being consequently of comparatively little value except to the most painstaking medical reader. We think that it will suffice for our purpose if we state in a few words the opinions which were held by the ancient physicians to the time of Galen, those found in the works of the Arabian physicians and the physicians of the middle ages, and lastly, give a short analysis of the views held by the moderns since the sixteenth century; and since the advance of knowledge during those periods has not been very great, we shall avoid wearying the reader by multiplying quotations.

The leading characteristics of these eras in the knowledge of the disease may be thus epitomized. The ancients confounded phthisis with other diseases, both of the lungs and other organs, attended by wasting, but were yet well acquainted with the disease as we see it at this day. The Arabian physicians and those of the middle ages adhered to the opinion of Hippocrates and Galen, and advanced no new views of the nature of the disease; whilst among the moderns there has been, with advance of time, a gradual limitation of the disease to a tubercular state of the lungs, attempts to describe tubercle, speculations as to its immediate origin, an examination of its relation to scrofula, a consideration as to whether phthisis be essentially a disease of the general system or of the lungs, and a desire to generalize the conditions which mark the consumptive patient. Besides these there have been in all ages disputations as to the relation of hæmoptysis to phthisis, the contagious character of phthisis, and the efficiency of various remedial agents.

THE ANCIENTS.

Hippocrates (fourth and fifth centuries B.C.) describes several forms of consumption under the heads of phthisis, phthoe, and empyema, and mentions tubercle of the lungs, but he does not regard the tuberculous state of those organs as the essential condition of the disease. His description of a true phthisical case, as the disease is now regarded, is, however, very clear and decided. He includes also such diseases of the lungs as pleurisy and empyema. In a second form he also includes bronchitis, remitting during the summer; and in a third, scrofulous diseases of the spine. In reference to the cause of the disease he considers that the first form, which includes true phthisis, arises from hæmoptysis, and begins with a kind of catarrh, in which acrid matters descend from the head and cause ulceration of the lungs. He affirms that the expectoration in phthisis arises from ulcerations of the lungs, and he describes a test for pus which has held its ground until modern days; but expectorated matters in general were considered to descend from the head. The treatment of the disease may, in its broad outlines, be regarded as that adopted at the present day, viz., the free use of milk, whether asses', mares', goats', or cows' milk, when there was not much fever or headache, a moderate quantity of meat, fat fish, and other fats, with walking exercise for many miles daily, and the avoidance of changes of temperature.

The small portion of the works of *Aretæus* (second century) which has been preserved is quite inadequate to inform us as to the views of that great master of the art, but the following description of the general evidences of phthisis is as truthful and life-like as any which have been placed upon record:—

" There is present, weight in the chest (for the lungs are insensible to pain), anxiety, discomfort, loss of appetite; in the evening coldness, and heat towards morning; sweat more intolerable than the heat as far as the chest: expectoration varied as I have described." . . . . " Voice hoarse; neck slightly bent, tender, not flexible, somewhat extended; fingers slender, but joints thick; of the bones alone the figure remains, for the fleshy parts are wasted; the nails of the fingers crooked, their pulps are shrivelled and flat, for, owing to the flesh, they neither retain their tension nor rotundity; and owing to the same cause, the nails are bent, namely, because it is the compact flesh at their points which is intended as a support to them; and the tension thereof is like that of the solids. Nose sharp, slender; cheeks prominent and red; eyes hollow, brilliant and glittering; swollen, pale, or livid in the countenance; the slender parts of the jaws rest in the teeth as if smiling; otherwise of a cadaverous aspect. So also in all other respects; slender, without flesh; the muscles of the arms imperceptible; not a vestige of the mammæ, the nipples only to be seen; one may not only count the ribs themselves, but also easily trace them to their termination; for even the articulations at the vertebræ are quite visible, and their connections with the sternum are also manifest; the intercostal spaces are hollow and rhomboidal, agreeably to the configuration of the bone; hypochondriac region lank and retracted; the abdomen and flanks contiguous to the spine; joints clearly developed; prominent, devoid of flesh, so also with the tibia, ischium and humerus; the spine of the vertebræ, formerly hollow, now protrudes, the muscles on either side being wasted; the whole shoulder blades apparent, like the wings of a bird. If in these cases disorder of the bowels supervene, they are in a hopeless state.''

As he had taken Hippocrates for his model, was a man of acute observation, and lived several centuries later than his master, it may appear strange that he does not refer to tuberculous disease of the lungs in connection with phthisis, but we are not thence entitled to affirm that he was unacquainted with that condition. He also confounds phthisis with other diseases. In the treatment of the disease he particularly recommends sea voyages and the free use of milk and eggs.

Galen, a contemporary of Arctæus, adopted the view of the Greek physicians, that hectic fever and phthisis were not the same diseases, but he considered them to be so connected that consumption or marasmus occurs in the second stage of hectic. He evidently knew that hectic fever occurred with other diseases than consumption, and also that it was associated with the latter disease. In his view the disease might be due to an affection of the lungs or of other parts of the body, but when it was a true marasmus he regarded it as incurable. In reference to its cause he affirms that it is due to want of moisture, and that it is a drying up of the body, but it is probable that under this description he simply indicated the slow emaciation which is the constant characteristic of the disease. He, and others, had noticed the expectoration of calculous concretions in the sputa, and made the important observation—which needs to be repeated now—that bleeding from the fauces may be mistaken for bleeding from the lungs, as an indication of the existence or the progress of phthisis. In treatment he recommends asses', goats', cows', and human milk.

We do not stay to refer to the statements of *Aristotle, Dioscorides,* or *Celsus,* since whilst the first held strong views as to the contagiousness of the disease, the second gave much attention to treatment, and the third described with great care the symptoms and treatment of the disease, including the use of mutton suet boiled with flour, and the relation of hæmoptysis and catarrhal secretion, their views are represented by the authors already quoted.

Hence the general expression of the ancient views upon this subject is that the physicians well knew of the existence of true phthisis; they recognized the existence of tubercle, but did not associate the two conditions as belonging to the same disease; they doubtless included other deposits with those of tubercle, and included many diseases both of the lungs and general system with phthisis; they also believed that hæmoptysis was commonly a cause of phthisis, that catarrh preceded the attack, and that the proper treatment of the disease was by the improvement of the nutrition of the system by milk, flesh, meat, fat, exercise, and sea air.

THE MIDDLE AGES.

The views of the physicians from the time of Galen to the sixteenth or seventeenth century were essentially those of the earlier period, and we cannot find any decided advance in the knowledge of the disease if we except perhaps the views of *Alexander Trallian*, who called especial attention to the existence of tubercle of the lungs, and showed that its presence is followed by dyspnœa, and this by cough and the expectoration of a secretion generally viscid, but sometimes containing a calculus so hard as to cause a sound when it is spat upon a resisting surface. *Paulus Ægineta* treats of both hectic fever and consumption in cases of suppuration of the chest, and also mentions the expectoration of calculi; and in this respect the writings of *Avicenna* and *Forestus* agree. The Arabian physicians in general, with *Paracelsus, Oribasius, Aëtius*, and other distinguished men of those days, followed the Hippocratian doctrines. The two latter, *Avicenna* and *Forestus*, attached great importance to the use of the milk of various animals. *Avicenna* recommended a dry air, *Forestus*, discountenanced the arrest of hæmoptysis, *Capivaccius* gave sulphuric acid to cleanse the ulcers of the lungs, and *Avenzoar* advised the free use of olive oil in the treatment of the disease.

Hence the merit of the middle ages in reference to this department of medicine was the same as was due to them in general knowledge—that they kept and handed down to succeeding ages the knowledge of the early fathers, but being bound down by the authority of previous ages, they did not pursue investigations calculated to the increase of knowledge.

THE MODERNS TO THE TIME OF DR. BAILLIE.

In considering the views entertained by the physicians of the seventeenth and later centuries, we may divide them into those of two eras, with the line of separation drawn at the period of the publication of Dr. Baillie's researches on tubercle. This, however, must be regarded merely as a matter of convenience, and not as indicating that the line separates two well-defined classes of opinions: for whilst it is true that careful investigation of tubercle may date from the time of Baillie, it is also true that increasing importance was attached to the subject as the seventeenth passed into the eighteenth century. Indeed, in this, as in all other kinds of knowledge, improvement was gradual, until a period arrived when an observer having increased knowledge rapidly, utilized the speculations and labours of his predecessors, and became the representative of a class of opinions.

Of the numerous writers who preceded Baillie we must select Bennet, Desault, and Tralles, as representatives of the class who began to be aware of the essential connection which exists between a tubercular condition of the lungs and phthisis, although not without the admission that consumption might exist without disease of the lungs.

Bennet dissociated catarrh from phthisis, and showed that the secretion proceeds from the lungs primarily, and does not descend from the head. He accurately described the symptoms of true phthisis, and yet believed that consumption might occur when the lungs were sound. He also regarded hæmoptysis as a cause of the disease.

Morton adopted similar views as to the distinction between catarrh and consumption, and described the symptoms of the latter very accurately. He considered that there was a form of consumption of an asthmatic kind.

Desault had very clear views of the true connection between tubercle and phthisis, and believed that generally hæmoptysis occurs subsequently to the tubercle, and in this latter opinion he was supported by *Mudge* and *Gilchrist*. The ulceration of the lungs was known to be an effect and not a cause of the disease. He drew attention to the frequency with which disorders of the liver attend consumption, and held to the doctrine that the latter is a contagious disease. In his opinion the beneficial effect of exercise was by breaking down the tubercle.

Tralles expressly believed that tubercle was the immediate cause of consumption.

Stark described tubercle and vomicæ with much minuteness, and stated that he had found them in the cellular membrane. His views were an advance upon those previously held.

Portal divided phthisis into several varieties, and believed that there were three kinds of tubercles.

Pearson published in the "Philosophical Transactions" a series of minute inquiries into the character and composition of different kinds of expectoration.

VIEWS RESPECTING TUBERCLE.

The views of tubercle as found in the lungs are very various, and deserving of attention.

Sylvius regarded them as glands in the lungs which suppurate and form vomicæ. *Tralles* considered them to be bronchial glands and vesicles distended by humours. *Clayton* injected the veins of a dog with mercury, and found minute suppurations in the lungs, having each a globule of mercury at its centre. This was believed to indicate the mode of formation of tubercle. *Willis* was of opinion that the expectoration in phthisis proceeded from the minute vessels of the trachea, and was derived from the serous parts of the blood. When retained it putrified and formed ulcers. *Boerhaave* considered consumption to be a conversion of all the blood and chyle into pus. *Thomas Reid* believed that tubercle consists of obstruction of the exhalant vessels, caused by the viscidity of their contents. *Sydenham* divided consumption into four kinds, and in reference to the first—which includes cases of true phthisis—he states that the lungs, being incapable of assimilating the proper aliment, are overwhelmed with a crude phlegm, and that a part of the humours which ought to be thrown off by perspiration is retained by the lungs. *Rush* believed tubercle to be a collection of inorganic mucous substance. On considering these various opinions of the nature of tubercle, we cannot avoid seeing the similarity between some of them and those recently promulgated, and then withdrawn by Rokitansky, based upon the chemical learning of our day, which affirmed that the albuminous matters of the blood were expended in the formation of tubercle. The connection between scrofula and phthisis which was held to exist by those above-mentioned, who regarded tubercle as a gland, was generally maintained, and particularly by *Brillouet* in 1789, and *Radcliffe* (the latter at least believing it to be so in cold climates), and also by the Edinburgh school in general. On the other hand *Simmons*, in 1780, denied the connection both of phthisis and scrofula, and of tubercles and scrofulous glands.

AGE.

The age at which this disease prevails was the same two thousand years ago as now, for Hippocrates informs us that in his day it was from eighteen to thirty-five years.

CAUSES.

In reference to the assigned causes of the disease which were held up to this period, we may first cite catarrh, to which reference has been already made, and acrid humours, either generated in the lungs, or descending from the head, and produced no doubt by the catarrh, as held by *Sennertus*, and *Hoffmann*, and by *Huxham*, in 1758, when tubercles had been previously formed. *Borelli* believed that the smoke from the wicks of candles, and fat and oil when poured into a confined space and inhaled, was a cause of phthisis. *Spigelius* affirmed that in England it was commonly caused by tight dresses; whilst *Van Swieten* was of opinion that it was produced by the excess of animal food in which Englishmen indulged. *Stahl* agreed with the latter in believing that it was often due to inactivity and full living. *Sims* thought it to be frequently caused by the retention in the body of morbid matters produced by syphilis and gonorrhœa. *Avicenna* remarked upon the greater prevalence of phthisis in cold countries, and *Blane* affirmed it to be less frequent in hot climates. *Rush* associated the disease with civilization, for he remarked that it was unknown to the North American Indians before they associated with white men, and was not found among colonists in the earliest stage of civilization. *Walker*, speaking of the atrophy of nurses, attributed that disease to the use of tea in the place of food. *Musgrave* saw a connection between gout and consumption. *Withering* remarked that hostlers and grooms living in the alkaline air of the stable were rarely consumptive; and *De Haen* noticed the arrest of phthisis doing pregnancy.

CONNECTION WITH HECTIC AND HÆMOPTYSIS.

The connection of consumption with hectic fever has been already referred to. Amongst the Greeks, the two conditions were held to be distinct, except so far that consumption appeared in the course of hectic fever; but in later times the hectic came to be regarded as a cause of consumption. *Bontius* recognized a true consumption with hectic. *Macbride* regarded phthisis and tabes as the principal species of hectic fever, but yet he admitted that the symptoms of phthisis precede the hectic. *Cullen* defined consumption as an expectoration of purulent matter with a hectic fever, more or less exquisitely formed, and commonly with ulceration.

In reference to the connection of phthisis and hæmoptysis, it has been shown that the early fathers regarded the latter as a cause of the former, and this view has been shared by many moderns. *Cullen* states that "the consequence of hæmoptysis is phthisis," and *Hoffmann* asserts that half the cases arise from hæmoptysis; but *Desault*, *Mudge* (who believed it to be the consequence of obstruction in the lung), and *Gilchrist* affirmed it to result from, or at least to follow the deposition of tubercle. We have noticed the observation of *Galen* as to the occurrence of faucial hemorrhage, and *Van Swieten* believed that hemorrhage from the palate might be mistaken for tubercular hemorrhage.

CONTAGION.

The contagious nature of the disease was perhaps universally believed by the ancients, and the belief has been conveyed through later ages to our own times. *Sylvius*, *Hoffmann*, *Desault*, *Van Swieten*, and *Darwin* adopted it, and so much impressed were *Morgagni* and *Valsalva* with this quality of propagation that they declined to open the bodies of consumptive patients, and thus excused themselves for their inability to determine the immediate seat of tubercular deposition. *Portal* denied the contagious nature of the disease.

NATURE.

In reference to the nature of the disease in the sense of phthisis, as now understood, we have seen that it was regarded by the ancients as an ulceration of the lung; then there was a connection perceived between tubercle and phthisis; and then, as at the era of *Stark* or *Desault*, tubercle was regarded as having an essential connection with phthisis, but *Rush* maintained that phthisis was not essentially a disease of the lung, but an affection of the general system, and primarily a disease of debility. It may be questioned as to how far those who regarded it as a hectic fever believed it to be essentially a disease of the lung, and indeed many such writers affirmed that consumption might exist, and yet the lungs be sound.

TREATMENT.

We do not purpose to give an analysis of the methods of treatment which have been proposed, but shall be content to make a few observations only. Milk has been recommended in all ages with singular concurrence, and with enthusiasm by *Aretæus*, if we may judge by the list of good effects which he ascribes to it; but *Gideon Harvey* sneered at it, since he considered that it was to affect the disease by being directly applied to the cavity of the lungs. He, however, admitted that its fatty particles might possibly puff up those who swallow it into some degree of corpulency. *Mead* also attached less value to it than was the practice with other physicians of his day. Numerous physicians, as *Fr. Hoffmann*, added lime water to the milk. Eggs, meat, and fish were commonly recommended. Olive oil was commended by *Avenzoar*, fat by *Hippocrates*, mutton suet by *Celsus*. Sea voyaging was advised by *Aretæus* and the early physicians, but not by them universally. *Carmichael Smyth*, in modern times regarded it as prejudicial, and *Gilchrist* greatly approved it. Exertion in the open air was insisted upon by *Hippocrates*, who commended walking ten to fifteen miles a day; and in the middle ages and modern times, physicians have recommended their patients to become coachmen, in order to spend their time in the open air. Horse exercise has been commended in all ages, and in modern times by *Sydenham, Fuller, Mead, Gilchrist, Pringle, Van Swieten,* &c. *Carmichael Smyth* recommended swinging, which, he said, lowered the pulsation ten beats per minute. *Reid* recommended persons in phthisis to live in cow houses. Steel was employed in the middle ages, and bark in cases of hæmoptysis in modern times, by *Morton* and *Mead*, before the lungs had become ulcerated. *Fothergill*, recommended early abstinence, milk, vegetables, quiet of mind, good hours, moderate exercise, and change of scene. Counter-irritation by caustics was practised by *Hippocrates* and *Aretæus*, and by the actual cautery by *Galen*, and the practice in some form has been common in all ages. Sulphuric acid was employed in the middle ages with a view to its supposed local action upon the ulcers. Speaking with a loud voice was commended by *Sanctorius*. Bleeding was practised in all the periods under examination by a certain number of physicians. In modern times it has been enjoined by *Gideon Harvey, Pringle*, &c., but *Bartholin* found the heart thin and dry, or, in other words, fatty and shrunken, and but little blood in the body, and *Cheyne* remarked that the quantity of blood was much diminished in hectic fever. *Gideon Harvey*, besides bleeding, recommended the use of steel, opiates, and astringents.

At the end of the eighteenth century many physicians practised inhalation of various gases and vapours in the treatment of tubercular phthisis, amongst whom we may mention *Mudge, Fourcroy*, and *Beddoes*. *Fourcroy* observed the effects of the inhalation of oxygen, and found that it accelerated the pulse and respiration, and increased inflammatory action, and hence he regarded it as inimical to phthisis. *Beddoes*, whose work is a monument of industry, based his practice upon chemical theories, and arrived at the conclusion that in phthisis there is an excess of oxygen in the system, and consequently that free air was injurious to the patient. All these ideas tended to the belief that the inhalation of air containing carbonic acid was the proper plan of treatment. In our day, we see this theory of hyper-oxidation revived by Liebig, and also upon chemical grounds, and the recommendation that in phthisis the respiratory action should be lessened.

OPINIONS OF OUR OWN DAY.

We will now offer a few remarks upon the opinions which have been held since the time of Baillie, and endeavour to state those of distinguished men up to our own day upon some of the more important questions which have already been discussed.

Baillie, Bayle, Laennec, and *Carswell* gave a great impulse to researches into the nature of tubercle, and have brought down the knowledge almost to the present time. *Baillie* describes with great minuteness the physical characters of tubercles, and affirms that they are found in the cellular tissue, are not glandular and are not derived from the mucous follicles of the bronchia, but that they are minute at first, and increase in size; are firm, then curdy, and are converted into capsules containing a fluid, and occasionally they unite and form abscesses. In some cases they are diffused through the lungs. *Bayle* affirmed most distinctly that there is an essential relation between phthisis and the state of the lung, whatever may be the general symptoms. He divided phthisis into six species, and named them tubercular, granular, melanotic, ulcerous, calculous, and cancerous, and thereby included many deposits which have not lately been regarded as tubercle. He affirmed that there is a bloodvessel in every tubercle, and that the ulcerations are always lined by a membrane; but the expectoration is chiefly derived from the bronchial mucous membrane. He added a fourth stage to phthisis, which he called occult, because there was disease in the lung without any obvious symptom.

Laennec regarded tubercle as an accidental production, or a substance foreign to the natural organization of the lungs. He restricted phthisis absolutely to the tubercular disease, but with a slight recognition of a phthisis nervosa, and a form of chronic catarrh simulating tubercular phthisis. He divided or accepted the division of the tubercles into two principal forms, the insulated bodies, subdivided into miliary, crude, granular, and encysted, and the interstitial injection or infiltration with the three varieties, irregular, gray, and yellow. The miliary form is the most common, whilst the granular and encysted forms of Bayle are rare. He doubted if a bloodvessel were generally, much less always, present in the centre of a tubercle. He distinguished six stages of tubercle, viz., semi-transparent granulations, yellow and opaque at the centre, yellow and opaque throughout, but yet firm, gray infiltration chiefly around cavities, softened at the centre, and excavations; and he states that in the same lung two or three successive eruptions may be found. *Louis* substantially adopted the views of Laennec, and even more than the latter agreed with those of Bayle, and all affirmed that the apices of the lungs were especially liable to this deposit.

Dr. Carswell, in 1838, called attention to the important fact that tubercle is not usually found in the cellular tissue of organs, but, in the vast proportion of cases, *upon* mucous surfaces, and, as a general expression, *upon* the secreting surface of hollow organs. He affirmed that the gray semi-transparent substance did not necessarily precede the formation of the pale-yellow or opaque tubercular matter. The latter is found in but few organs, whilst the former is found in the air-cells and the serous membrane. It is without organization; but in the cow and other animals it assumes a concentric or laminated form, from the presence of albumen and fibrin. It is composed in men of albumen, fibrin, and gelatine, and softens from the circumference, and not from the centre.

Subsequent to this period the microscope has been more particularly employed in determining the precise nature of tubercle, and certain cellular and granular elements have been found in the deposit.

In 1816, *Laennec* commenced the series of researches which led to his system of Mediate Auscultation, and which must be regarded as the most important discovery in medical science of this century. Not that he, in truth, was the first to make some use of the ear to ascertain the state of the chest, for *Hippocrates* did the same, to a limited extent, and *Avenbrugger* to a much greater degree; but for all that has rendered knowledge upon this subject exact, and built up into a science, we are indebted to Laennec. The signs, and consequently the diagnosis of phthisis, and the knowledge of its progress, and therefore the prognosis, became more exact from his labours.

Louis followed in the same path, and gave a more accurate detail of the symptoms, etiology, and pathology of the disease than any who had preceded him.

M. Piorry has, at various times, expressed novel and independent views both as to the nature and the treatment of phthisis ; and in a paper recently read before the *Académie de Médecine*, he developed the following propositions :—

" 1. Pulmonary Phthisis is a combination of multifarious variable phenomena, and not a morbid unity ; 2. Hence there does not and cannot exist a specific medicine against it ; 3. Therefore, neither iodine nor its tincture, neither chlorine nor sea salt, nor tar, can be considered in the light of anti-phthisical remedies ; 4. There are no specifics against phthisis, but there are systems of treatment to be followed in order to conquer the pathological states which constitute the disorders ; 5. In order to cure consumptive patients, the peculiar affections under which they labour must be studied and appreciated, and counteracted by appropriate means ; 6. The tubercle cannot be cured by the use of any remedy, but good hygienic precautions may prevent its development ; 7. The real way to relieve, cure, or prolong the life of consumptive patients, is to treat their various pathological states, which ought to receive different names according to their nature ; 8. Consumption thus treated has often been cured, and oftener still, life has been considerably prolonged ; 9. Phthisis should never be left to itself, but always treated as stated above ; 10. The old methods, founded on the general idea of a single illness called phthisis, are neither scientific nor rational, &c. ; 11. The exact and methodical diagnosis of the various pathological states which constitute the malady, will dictate the most useful treatment for it."

The most remarkable features in the treatment of the disease during the present century have been, the removal of the patient to a milder climate, and the administration of cod-liver oil. The former was advised in all stages of the disease, and seemed to be called for by the urgency of the cough, and perhaps by the frequent presence of inflammatory complications. Hence multitudes were sent away to die distant from their home and friends. This evil has been abated of late years, and care is now taken to avoid such a recommendation when the disease is far advanced and the life is in peril. The latter is of very recent introduction into general use—only since the commencement of the career of the distinguished Professor of the Institutes of Medicine in Edinburgh ; but, as a remedy in other diseases, it had been recommended and adopted to a small degree at the end of the last century. During the last fifteen years its use has been universal, in all stages of phthisis, and in many other diseases.

SUMMARY.

Having thus sketched the progress of opinion and knowledge upon this subject, let us, by way of summary, endeavour to show in what degree the knowledge of the present day differs from that of preceding ages :—

1. The diseases formerly included in the term Phthisis or Consumption were found to be various, and one class has been selected out from the number, and the term rigorously restricted to it.

2. Tubercle in the lungs is regarded as the distinctive mark of this class.

3. The term tubercle formerly included numerous deposits, varying in nature and character ; but now it is, as far as possible, restricted to one kind of deposit.

4. The increase of the means of investigation has opened new difficulties in determining the nature of deposits, because the new kind of knowledge is yet imperfect ; and hence the nature of tubercle has not been settled on its histological characters.

5. The question of the essential identity of scrofula and phthisis is yet undecided.

6. The intimate nature of phthisis, as to whether its first origin lies in the lungs or in the general system, is still undecided.

7. The immediate source of the deposit found in the lungs is still undetermined.

8. The occurrence of the deposit is generally still held to be the first evidence of the existence of the disease.

9. The existence of the deposit and its nature, the progress of the deposition in the lungs, and the site, degree, and progress of the destruction of those organs, is a knowledge perhaps peculiar to this century, and is now in a highly advanced state.

10. The state of the general system was as well known to the ancients as to ourselves, if we select those cases known to the former which are now alone admitted by the latter.

11. The fatal tendency of the disease has been in all ages alike admitted, and at this day nearly one-eighth of the whole mortality in England is due to this now carefully selected class of cases.

12. There is an impression that, within a few years, the effect of modern treatment has been to prolong life during the attack of the disease; and our distinguished colleague, Dr. Williams, has felt himself justified in saying how long it is increased. There are also grounds for believing that a cure is sometimes effected ; but the mortality referred to, and the general feeling of professional and non-professional people alike, is that the disease is a fatal one.

15. The general principles of treatment and the methods employed are still the same as in former ages (due allowance being made for the separation of the particular class of cases which we are now able to effect), except that now bleeding is not resorted to, and

the connection with catarrh is not necessarily admitted, although we fully admit the influence of a cold in developing the disease. That there has been a change in the aspect of the disease at various eras is highly probable, according to the habits and prevailing constitution of the age, and hence the former practice and views might then have been as little incorrect as ours are now.

16. There has been but little variation in the remedies employed in all ages, as we have seen that milk, cream, eggs, meat, vegetables, exercise, open air, sea voyaging, change of climate, and adaptation of temperature and dryness of the air, steel, bark, olive oil, mutton suet, &c., have been heretofore employed. There have been the selection and rejection of minor remedies as emetics, digitalis, hydrocyanic acid, &c., with every age, and the leading treatment of this day has been anticipated, although not in the precise form of cod-liver oil.

17. Hence as a final expression we may state that, whilst we have a selected class of cases, with an improved diagnosis and pathology, and these improved views are so largely shared by all practitioners, that the treatment is now similar in all parts of the kingdom, we are not agreed as to the essential nature of the disease, have no unfailing mode of treatment, and the disease is still essentially and almost as universally a fatal one as it has been in all ages.

CHAPTER III.

HISTORICAL SKETCH AS TO THE VIEWS ON THE EARLY STAGE OF PHTHISIS.

In the foregoing historical sketch we have always referred to phthisis as a disease commencing with the deposition of tubercles in the lungs, and its fatal character and progressive changes in the lungs apply to the disease when so considered. But there has been, at least in recent years, a belief that there are conditions existing anterior to this deposit which have such a connection with phthisis, that, if continued, the deposition in the lungs commonly appears. These have not been regarded necessarily as cause and effect, but as pre-existent circumstances, having a general tendency to the sequence just pointed out, and have commonly been designated "predisposing causes," and whether that or the term "first stage of phthisis," would the most correctly indicate them, will depend upon the view which is taken of their causative influence. If it be shown that they have such a connection with the deposition of tubercle, that they are necessarily, or nearly so, pre-existent to the deposit, then we truly have a stage of the disease in which the conditions are quite different from those found after the deposition of tubercle, and to which the fatality of the later stage would not necessarily belong. This we consider one of the most important questions of the day, and worthy of the most serious and unbiassed consideration of medical men; for if there be such a stage, if it can be recognized, and if it be curable, then it follows that instead of our energies being wasted upon a comparatively hopeless task, we may find the highest of all rewards to which the physician can aspire—the saving of a countless multitude of lives. Hence we propose, before expressing our own views upon the subject, to adduce such testimony as the medical literature or experience of the present age will afford, and endeavour to determine its precise value upon this subject.

In pursuing this plan it is manifest that we cannot go back beyond the period of Laennec's discoveries, because until then there were not the means of determining the existence of tubercle with the exactitude which is now requisite, neither can we expect that Laennec or his contemporaries should give any response to our question, because they had established the separation of this class of cases by the very fact of tubercle being present in the lungs, and consequently, could not admit that the disease existed previously to the deposition of tubercles. Hence, from the works of *Bayle, Laennec, Andral*, and *Louis*, we learn only that there were sometimes conditions as diarrhœa, which preceded and led to the deposition of tubercle, and such designations as "irregular manifest phthisis," and "latent phthisis," concerning which it was stated either that the disease did not begin in the lungs, or that the evidence of disease of the lungs was entirely wanting, whilst the general symptoms were urgent.

Sir James Clark, in the preface to his admirable monograph,[1] especially calls attention to the state of the general system in which tuberculous disease of the lungs originates, and shows clearly that tubercle is a secondary condition resulting from a pre-existent state of the general system. He remarks that "the total inefficacy of all means hitherto adopted for diminishing the frequency or reducing the mortality of this class of diseases is of itself sufficient incitement to us to seek for some other method of remedying the evil; and it is evident to me that this can only be done, with any reasonable prospect of success, by directing the attention to such measures as are calculated to prevent the hereditary transmission of the particular morbid state in which the primal disease originates, and to correct the predisposition to it in infancy and youth." In the introduction he further remarks that the views of Laennec "have tended to keep up the idea that consumption is a local disease referable to a local cause, and thus the investigation of the constitutional origin of tubercles, by far the most important part of the subject,

---

[1] Treatise on Pulmonary Consumption, &c.

has been neglected." "We must carry our researches beyond the pulmonary disease which is only a secondary affection, the consequence of a pre-existing constitutional disorder; the necessary condition which determines the production of tubercles." "That which is considered the early is in reality the advanced stage of the disease, and that tubercle is a secondary affection originating in a peculiar morbid condition of the system." "If the labour and ingenuity which have been misapplied in fruitless attempts to cure an irremediable condition of the lungs had been rightly directed to the investigation of the causes and nature of tubercular disease, the subject of our inquiry would have been regarded in a very different light from that in which it is at the present period." Sir James strongly held the view that there is a diathesis allied to the scrofulous in which the disease originates, and his aim was so to improve the general system that tubercular disease in the lungs should not appear.

Dr. Barlow writes:[1] "The stage of deposition, which is often regarded as the first, is that in which tubercles are first present in the lungs, and as they are generally considered as essential to phthisis, it may, perhaps, appear illogical to speak of any previous state of disease; but setting aside this difficulty, as rather formal than real, it must be obvious that since tubercle is itself a pathological epigenesis or morbid product, there must have been some antecedent diseased action preceding or even causing this product. This previous marked condition is of a twofold character—the one generally affecting the whole system, constituting what has been already described as the tubercular diathesis, and the other local, depending upon a determination of blood to the lungs."

Dr. Hughes Bennett remarks:[2] "Phthisis in its incipient stage may be considered a very curable disease, indeed so much so, that cure is, as we have seen, spontaneously accomplished by nature in a vast number of cases."

Dr. Hamilton Roe, our senior colleague, has kindly expressed to us his opinion upon this subject in the following words: "Consumption never attacks any one until his health is broken down, and therefore it must be preceded by the ordinary signs of cachectic condition, and though few or any of them are so characteristic of any particular complaint that they may not be the forerunners of some other, they are so very frequently followed by phthisis, that wherever they appear we have cause to apprehend that it is approaching. The signs which first attract observation, and which gradually become more marked, are, an altered expression of the countenance, an unusually faded colour of the face and skin generally, that differs from anæmia, a look of languor, debility and depression of spirits, and dulness of the eyes. On inquiry, we learn that a degree of exertion which at one time was not felt at all inconveniently, now produces fatigue;

---

[1] Manual of Practice of Medicine.   [2] Pulmonary Consumption, 1859.

that going up stairs causes breathlessness and disturbance of the
heart's action ; that the appetite is capricious, and plain food un-
palatable ; that symptoms of indigestion are manifested ; that sleep
is not sound as usual, and that the patient wakes in the morning
unrefreshed ; that the temper is irritable, and the pulse feeble."

Dr. Richard Quain has also courteously communicated to us the
following observations. Every day's clinical experience decides that
tubercles in the lungs are but the local manifestation of a morbid
process which has its origin elsewhere. What this process is, what
the exact seat of its origin, and why the lungs become the seat of
tubercles are some of the most important subjects to which investigation can be directed. Scientific research and clinical observation
have, within a few years, supplied many facts calculated to aid in
answering these inquiries ; and practical physicians have sought by
gaining " early information" of the féatures which characterize the
constitutional conditions, and of the physical signs which mark local
changes in the lungs, to anticipate the malady in its earliest stage,
and thus to check a progress, which, if allowed to continue, might
be impossible to impede. Enough has been gained to justify the
confident belief that much more is within reach of earnest inquiry.

Dr. Cotton,[1] under the general heading of " *The period preceding
the formation of tubercle*," states that, " sometimes this, which we
may term the *preliminary stage*" (or dawn as he elsewhere terms
it), " is so well defined that to fail in recognizing it would be almost
inexcusable ; at other times it is either too brief or too indistinctly
marked to be detected." These symptoms are commonly, slow diminution of bodily vigour, good spirits, pallid or sallow complexion,
animated yet careworn expression of the features, hurried and anxious
movements, uncertain appetite, imperfect digestive power, and diarrhœa. Variable, but generally small and excitable pulse. Sleep
restless and occasional perspiration, and invariably loss of weight.
The duration of this stage is very variable. He also devotes a chapter to the " treatment of phthisis before tubercle is deposited."

Dr. Lawson[2] explicitly treats upon the symptoms and signs of the
precursory stage, and explains that " the phrase *precursory stage* is
designed to indicate a morbid state existing intermediately between
the mere diathesis on the one hand, and the deposit of solid tubercles
in the lungs on the other. The *diathesis* is a constitutional predisposition to disease, which, under favourable circumstances, may
never become developed ; the *precursory stage*, on the contrary, is
the beginning of a positive morbid action, which, if not arrested,
surely and steadily progresses to the deposit of tubercles." He
then divides the symptoms into those which refer to the state of the
general system, and " those which spring directly from the pulmonary organs and respiratory passages." Those which refer to the
state of the general system are, defective vital powers, impaired

---

[1] On Consumption.   [2] On Phthisis Pulmonalis, 1861.

strength, slight loss of weight, and lowness, and irregular action of the functions, chills and febricula from variable conditions of calorification and innervation, a state of debility of the heart, and arterial and capillary circulation, disease of the pharyngo-laryngeal structures in a large majority of cases, trivial cough and spitting, and perhaps a little hemorrhage.

The evidences furnished by the lungs are, debility of the moving parietes of the chest, with incomplete dilatation, but capability of perfect expansion on deep inspiration. The percussion note is less clear, and over a large area, from deficient mobility of the thorax ; and the respiratory murmur is generally (not partially) weak and jerking. He strongly asserts that these evidences, described by him in detail, are associated with the pretubercular period.

Mr. Ancell, in his laborious work on "Tuberculosis," states: "The inspiratory and expiratory motions being accelerated, but small, or small without being accelerated, indicate that the function of respiration, measured by the extent of these motions, is below the standard of health ; the frequency of motion by no means compensating for the loss of extent. It shows a diminution of the *vital capacity* or *breathing power* of the lungs, which occurs in tuberculosis before any deposit or appreciable organic disease in these organs."

Since 1855, we have called professional attention to this subject on numerous occasions, as in papers "On the Curable Stage of Phthisis," read before the Western Medical Society ; on "The Pre-Tubercular Stage of Phthisis," read before the Medical Society of London, and published in the "Edinburgh Medical and Surgical Journal," 1856 ; on the "Principles and Treatment of Phthisis," in the "Midland Quarterly Medical Journal," and since separately published ; and in a course of lectures on "Certain Views on the Nature and Treatment of Phthisis," delivered at the House for Consumption, &c., Brompton, and published in the "British Medical Journal," 1856–7, as well as in other papers since published in the same journal. In the paper on "The Principles and Treatment of Chronic Phthisis," we introduced the following observations on the evidences of the first or pre-tubercular stage: "Its own evidences are shorter breathing, less breath motion, feeble and shorter inspiratory sounds, and particularly the vesicular sounds ; and this may be more or less general over the whole of both lungs. Expiration, quick, forcible, and perfect. Deep inspiration may be effected, but it is not effected by the patient, unless at least, his attention be directed to the defect, and more commonly not until he has given attention by repeated efforts. This may be readily proved by the inspiration. The quantity of tidal air is often diminished in ordinary breathing ; the general indications of the body are those of atonicity, and possibly the rate of pulsation and respiration may be increased, and the complexion and condition of system evince a state of mal-nutrition. There will probably be flattening of the chest, depending upon original conformation, or upon the progress of the disease. The same remark will also apply to dulness on percussion. Cough may or

may not exist, as also some hæmoptysis. The essence of the whole
is less respiratory action, and as this varies in degree, extent, and
duration, so will the other signs vary."

In the discussion which followed the promulgation of these views,
and which appeared in the "Medical Times and Gazette," 1857, *Dr.
Markham* stated : "Of course we all know well enough that there
is a morbid condition of the body existing anterior to the deposit of
tubercle in the lungs ; that tubercle is not the disease, but merely
the external and tangible manifestation of that anterior condition—
perhaps the last of a long series of antecedent changes which have
been working in the system ; that the disease may be thus in the
body from the moment of the first evolution of the ovarian vesicle ;
and we know also that treatment is not directed to the tubercle,
but to the averting, it may be, of that morbid condition which pre-
sides over the deposition."

Such are the opinions which have been placed upon record as to
the existence of a precursory or pre-tubercular stage of phthisis.
For the reasons which we have already assigned, the numbers of
persons who could give testimony of the nature sought by us are
few; but in proportion as they have been educated at a period distant from that of the teaching of the Laennec school, and in proportion also as a spirit of inquiry has become more general, we
find those who entertain the view that there must be a condition of
the general system, or of the lung, or of both, which precedes and
leads to the deposit of tubercle. There are also many, and even
distinguished men, who have not sufficient belief in the efficiency of
auscultation to reveal the earliest deposition of tubercle, and who
will not admit that, although there are no evidences of the deposition, they are not entitled to affirm that the deposition does not
exist. This confidence, we are aware, presupposes the possession
of a degree of knowledge only to be attained by constant and large
experience in the careful examination of these cases; but for those
who possess it to hesitate in the mass of cases, to believe that
tubercle is absent when there are no evidences of its presence, implies, we think, a desire for a degree of evidence which is not
required in management of the ordinary concerns of life, and to
attach undue importance to the cases (very few in comparison with
the whole) in which small nodules of so-called tubercle have been
found after death, but neither discovered nor sought for during life.

We think that we may, with confidence, refer to the authorities
now adduced as proof of the advance which has been made on this
subject within the last few years ; and whilst they differ in opinion
as to the nature of this early stage, they all tend to prove that
there is a stage of the disease which exists before the deposition of
tubercle, and that its evidences are to be found both in the lungs
and the general system. We cannot but congratulate ourselves
that the views which we propounded seven years ago are almost
identical with those which so able a writer as Dr. Lawson has recently issued.

PART II.

NATURE AND EVIDENCES OF THE EARLY STAGE OF PHTHISIS.

CHAPTER IV.

GENERAL OBSERVATIONS.

HAVING thus concluded our sketch of the history of the disease, and shown how far an early stage has been heretofore recognized, we proceed to consider the nature and evidences of the latter, as a preliminary proceeding to a consideration of the treatment.

STAGES OF THE DISEASE.

It is customary at the present day to mark the progress of Phthisis by reference to the lungs only, and to divide it into three stages, of which the 1st is limited to the period of deposition of tubercle; the 2d includes softening of tubercle, and destruction of tissue, and the 3d is that period when a cavity exists. There would no doubt be defects in every arrangement which might be proposed, but we think that there is a radical defect in this one in the omission of all reference to the general system, and in separating the period of destruction of tissue from that of the formation of a cavity, which are evidently parts of the same process. The first has existed ever since the modern views were first established, but the latter was unknown to Laennec and Louis, for they recognized but two stages, those of consolidation and destruction. The existing arrangement has also the further defect of implying that the importance of the case increases in proportion as the stages advance, omitting all reference to the important facts of the greater or less extent of the lung disease, its limitation to one lung or otherwise, and the amount of injury inflicted upon the general system, whereas we know that so far is this from being necessarily true, that no adequate opinion can be formed of the condition of a case by indicating the stage in which the disease exists. Moreover, it has the defect of implying that the general tubercular condition is as exactly limited in its progress as the stage indicates, so that the deposition having proceeded

to a certain point, is arrested, and the work of destruction commences, and this at length ends in the 3d condition, in which the
softened matter is removed, and a vacant place or cavity is left, but
in truth all the actions proceed simultaneously in different parts of
the lungs in nearly every case, and whilst the agent of destruction
is busy in one part, new tubercle is being deposited in others. Hence
the basis of the classification is only valid when we fix the attention
upon one and the same restricted portion of the lungs. If relation
to the danger of life and the progress of the disease could be included in the grounds of classification, it is clear that the state of
the general system would take precedence of that of the lung, for
at all times it is the condition of the general system to which we refer
when we attempt to estimate the chances of impending danger.
The condition of the lungs is good ground for diagnosis, but that of
the system is the true ground for an *immediate* prognosis.

As our purpose in the following work is to limit the attention to
that state of the disease in which treatment is of the greatest avail,
we shall not enter further into the question of classification, but
shall content ourselves with indicating the division which we would
adopt. We divide the progress of the disease into three stages, the
1st including all the conditions existing before any evidence of the
deposition of tubercle is afforded ; the 2d the period of tubercular
deposition ; and the 3d that of destruction ; thus adopting the
earlier classification, with the addition of the pretubercular period
of the disease.

CO-EXISTENCE OF GENERAL AND LOCAL DISEASE.

We now purpose to consider the nature and the evidences of the
early stages of phthisis, and to show how far they may be distinguished both from the more advanced state of the disease, and
from other conditions with which the general evidences are allied,
and we hope to prove that the first stage has a substantive existence,
and presents features by which it may be readily recognized.

*The evidences of the first stage are associated both with the general
system and the lungs, and in both they are co-existent in time.*

In this part of the discussion it must be borne in mind that whilst
the lungs may be regarded as separate organs, with special duties
and responsibilities which cannot be delegated to other structures,
they are at the same time an important and essential part of the
general system.   Hence it is impossible that any morbid condition
of the lungs should long exist without inducing a diseased state of
the other functions of the body, which together constitute the general system ; neither is it likely that any continued diminution of the
general vital powers should occur without the lungs entering into
the community of suffering.   Strictly speaking, there must be a
period in acute conditions in which the one may be diseased whilst
the other is sound, but in chronic states, of which the prime moment

of departure from health cannot be ascertained, and in which the changes towards disease proceed slowly and insidiously, there is no period in which it may be safely affirmed that the one suffers whilst the other is free. Both alike are under the influence of general causes, and they suffer simultaneously, although it may be in very various degrees. Hence, whilst in the disease in question, we have a localized disease of the lungs, and such a variation of the general functions of the body as to represent a diminution of the vital powers, we can neither dissociate one from the other, nor assign a precedence in time to the one or the other. They are co-existent conditions, and react upon each other. It is therefore rather in this belief than with a view to prove a dependence of one upon the other, that we shall now proceed to consider in detail the conditions of the system generally, and of the lungs and other local organs in particular. Neither do we wish it to be understood that there is any clearly-defined line of demarcation between the lungs and the general system in their functional character, and it is only in their anatomical and physical relations that we shall consider them separately.

GENERAL EXPRESSION OF DISEASED ACTION.

With evidences derived from the many functions which constitute the general system, there must be a common expression, either as to the nature or the tendency of the changes induced.

It will be evident that no general changes can occur in the functions of the body without having debility as their issue. The due and harmonious working of the body constitutes health, and whilst there may be degrees of health, there can be no variation in the vital actions which shall exceed the condition known as health, for the most perfect functional condition is health. Whenever changes occur there must be a disturbance of the balance of the vital actions, and as a result, a condition of disease in that particular function which is primarily changed, and in the whole system of functions which is more or less dependent upon it. Derangement of function must, therefore, induce less vital power, or, in other words, less health; and, as a consequence, the system is less able to supply its own wants, and to defend itself against adverse influences, and debility or lessened vital power is established. Hence there are not any true general sthenic conditions, if the standard of health be regarded as our basis, since health is the natural condition of the system, and nothing stronger or higher in degree can occur; yet, if we compare healthy with diseased conditions, we find them relatively sthenic and asthenic; but the latter is essentially below, whilst the former cannot be above health. The general expression which we seek as indicative of the first stages of phthisis is asthenia or lessened vital power.

3

VARIATIONS OF THE TYPE OF HEALTH AND DISEASE.

The separate conditions, which together constitute the general expression, must be variable in degree as the type of health varies.

It is important to bear in mind that unless the type of health, as evidenced by the general organism be identical in all persons, the variations from that type cannot be universally the same. In our desire for simplicity and uniformity in the diagnosis and treatment of unhealthy conditions, we seek for general descriptions and directions which shall be an universal and infallible guide ; but as such a desire confounds all the varieties which nature has established, it is evident that it is the expression of limited knowledge. As we must admit the existence of various types of health, each having its own peculiarities, although all possess outlines in common, so when we consider changes from disease in their earliest manifestations, we are compelled to admit variations in its evidences, and must seek to classify them as we have already classified types of health under the heads of temperaments, races and climatic conditions, until the diseased changes have proceeded so far that they indicated the conditions upon which life itself depends, when they will assume aspects of greater similarity.

As we have in the first stage of phthisis the earlier deviations from a state of health, we must be prepared to admit much variation in the evidences of the disease, and yet not thence assume either that the disease is protean in its character or the description of it inexact. Moreover, as these conditions are common with others which are found in the course of other diseases, it must not be assumed that they have no definite relation to the one under discussion, for the general system may be similarly influenced, whilst other and local conditions may vary.

The sanguineo-nervous and the lymphatic may be regarded as the extreme types of temperament, as seen in this country.

By the sanguineo-nervous temperament we mean one in which there is great activity of the whole organism, as seen in the high flow of spirits, the excitable nervous system, rapidity of circulation and respiration, readiness for exertion, rapidity of digestion and transformation, and as externally marked by a body of medium development, a form a little given to rotundity, a coloured complexion, bright aspect, light coloured eyes, and hair varying in shade from brown through sandy and auburn to flaxen. The tendency of such a system is to excess of action, and therefore to waste.

The lymphatic temperament is represented by comparative inactivity of all the mental and vital actions. This is shown by slower mental appreciation, tendency to low spirits, soft and not rapid pulse. Feebler and slower respiration, lack of desire to make exertion, somewhat spare habit, or if fleshy, the flesh is loose and flabby ; assimilation slow and imperfect, eyes brown or dark, aspect dull, soft, pasty, and expressionless; complexion pale or sallow, and hair variable, from light brown to black. Such a system is deficient in the power of reproduction of tissue, and tends to exhaustion by failing to supply.

Without discussing this subject more minutely than our present purpose demands, it will, we believe, be admitted that the evidences of the early deviations from health must be very different in the two classes of cases, and the admixtures of them which abound in society; and that although in both alike the tendency of the system is to deficiency of vital power, that condition is brought about by very different means, requires very different modes of investigation, will vary greatly in the rate of downward progression, and offers very different chances of restoration to health.

There is no one temperament which is exclusively found in phthisical patients; but the two extreme types are largely diffused amongst them.

We have largely inquired into the relative frequency of these types of health, as seen in phthisical persons, at least so far as refers to the respectable class who are the out-patients at the Hospital for Consumption, and who represent the masses of the community. In this investigation we have determined the questions which are usually included in the idea of temperament; such as the colour of the hair, eyes, and complexion, the rotundity of the body, and the degree of excitability of the nervous system; and, in doing so, have expressly excluded the period during which the disease has existed, and have ascertained the natural or healthy conditions of the individuals. We will now cite the results in the order just given.

The Hair.—The variations of colour of the hair which we have recorded are black, chocolate, dark brown, brown, sandy, light brown, light, and flaxen; and in arranging the results of 1000 cases for analysis, we have taken the medium brown colour as the standard, and have compared the whole of the darker and lighter shades respectively with it. Of the whole number of cases, male and female, 82.1 per cent. exhibited the medium tint, whilst 34.7 per cent. had darker, and 30 per cent. light coloured hair.   The instances of the extreme colour were few, so that black hair was found in only 1.4; chocolate, in 5.7; sandy, in 4.1; and flaxen, or nearly white, in .38 per cent.; and hence the various shades of brown were almost universal. In reference to the influences of sex, we may remark that the medium and the darker colour were more frequent in the females, whilst the lighter greatly preponderated in the males. Thus, in reference to each of the three divisions, medium brown, dark, and light, the percentage of frequency in females was 34, 41, and 19, whilst in males it was 31, 30, and 38.   Black and sandy hair was, however, more frequently found in males than females.

The Eyes.—We recorded three colours only, viz., black, hazel, and gray, with the darker and lighter shades of the two latter, so that blue was included in the gray. The number of investigations was 1000, and of these 74.0 per cent. had gray eyes, 23.0 per cent. had hazel, and not 1 per cent. had black eyes, so that the preponderance of one colour was very marked. The gray colour prevailed in the men, and the hazel in the women; the percentage of the two colours being, in women 69 and 26, and in men 77 and 20.

The Complexion.—The colour of complexion in the phthisical patients is not that which had existed in the same person in health, but we found no difficulty in ascertaining whether the natural tint of the complexion had been coloured or pale, and the replies of 1000 persons were arranged under these two heads. The coloured complexion was found in 58.3, and the pale in 40 per cent. There was also a considerable preponderance of the florid complexion in females over males, whilst the pale was noticed reversely in nearly an equal proportion. The actual frequency was: florid, 65 per cent. females, and 53 per cent. males; pale, 34 per cent. females, and 44 per cent. males.

The Habit of Body.—The inquiries were made from 1000 patients under the four heads of rounded, spare, muscular, and bony; but for this analysis we have arranged the answers under two only, viz., fleshy and spare. The general returns showed singular equality, for 45.8 were fleshy, and 51.9 per cent. were naturally spare; but there was a marked difference in the two sexes, since 60 per cent. of the women had been fleshy, and 37 per cent. spare, whilst of the men 33 per cent. only had been fleshy, and 61 per cent. had been spare.

The Degree of Excitability.—We sought to elicit this fact by ascertaining if in good health the patients had exhibited evidences of an excitable, firm, or languid temperament, and as the first greatly preponderated, it will suffice if we quote the returns. Of 1000 persons, 71 per cent. exhibited the excitable or susceptible temperament, and the proportion was nearly equally distributed in the two sexes, since in females it was 75, and in males 68 per cent.

We have thus endeavoured to epitomize the results of this part of a very laborious inquiry into the etiology of phthisis, to which we shall have to recur on numerous occasions. As a general expression of the whole, it may be stated that there is the greatest diversity in all the points of inquiry in phthisical persons in this country, but there is a preponderance of cases with gray eyes, florid complexion, fleshy habit of body, and excitability of temperament. Whether, however, they differ in these respects from the community at large has not yet been determined. In reference to the sexes, the females constituted the greater proportion of the cases with dark hair, hazel eyes, florid complexion, and fleshy habit, whilst there was much equality in reference to pale complexions and excitability of temperament.

In the following chapters we shall consider the state of the several functions of the body in the two classes of cases just indicated, and shall have occasion sometimes to refer to them separately.

CHAPTER V.

MENTAL AND NERVOUS ORGANIZATION.

THE general condition of the nervous system in the sanguineous cases is marked by sensibility and excitability. The spirits are greatly elated under pleasing circumstances, so that the vivacity is beyond that of health, whilst at other times there is sudden and unaccountable depression, rapidly alternating with the former, and becoming more marked by contrast. The elation is chiefly found after the breakfast hour and until the afternoon, whilst the depression follows fatigue, precedes the meals, and is common in the evening and the early morning, before and at the hour of rising. In the middle hours of the day the spirits readily answer every call, but in the evening they are not only low, but they do not readily obey the impulses which at other periods excite them.

The same remarks also apply to the general nervous organism so far as relates to its increased excitability, for it is unusually sensitive to all impressions, whether pleasing or painful. The influence of sudden impressions, whether of mental emotions or of physical occurrences, is increased, so that shock, whether of the mental or general nervous organism, is more easily induced. Fear more certainly paralyzes, pleasure exhilarates, pain exhausts, and cold revulses than under ordinary conditions. The influence of the period of the day is different from that which is found in reference to the spirits, for the increased excitability is the greatest in the evening, night, and early morning, and the body is then the most liable to be injured by adverse agencies.

If we now turn to the patients of a lymphatic temperament, we commonly find that the spirits are depressed under all conditions, and at every period of the day, whilst the degree of sensibility of the general organism remains unchanged.

Hence in a large number of cases it will be found that there is much diversity in the sensitiveness of the mental and general organization ; and when we add to this the influence of the events of life upon the masses of the community, we shall readily admit that, whilst there may be much diversity in degree, there will be great uniformity in the occurrence of the fact of depressed spirits and disturbance of the general sensibility.

CHAPTER VI.

ALIMENTATION.

The whole of the processes concerned in the function of alimentation are commonly lessened in vigour.

This proposition we believe to have the widest application, and yet at the same time to have only a limited force.

APPETITE.

The appetite seldom remains natural, but is somewhat lessened in respect of food in general and of some foods in particular, and is commonly wayward and uncertain.

There are, doubtless, many cases in which no noticeable change of the appetite has occurred, for, since men usually take more food than they strictly need, and the appetite falls into a routine course, there may be a certain diminution in and variation of it before the change is noticed, but we venture to affirm that on careful inquiry it will be admitted that the appetite is not so good as was formerly the case. The period of the day when it is in the greatest defect is the morning.

Whilst pursuing an inquiry into certain circumstances met with in phthisical patients, we thought it would be of interest to ascertain in what degree the ordinary articles of diet were disliked by phthisical patients before their disease commenced, in the hope that by the aid of a similar inquiry to be made upon healthy persons we might determine if there were any constitutional peculiarities in this respect in this large class of persons. This investigation is incomplete, but we have abstracted the returns from about 400 patients, of whom 276 were cases of phthisis. The inquiry included acids, sugar, tea, coffee, vegetables, fruits, bread, meat, milk, and fat, and the question was asked whether they had liked or disliked them in health. The combinations of so large a series precludes the possibility of giving the results in detail, but we shall quote the principal facts which have been obtained.

The number of cases in which one of the articles was the sole food disliked were few, except in reference to fat, viz.: acids, 2.1; sugar, 2.8; tea, .7; coffee, 2; vegetables, .3; fruits, 1; bread, .7; meat, .3; and fat, 23.4 per cent., and there was not an instance in which milk was solely objected to.

When, however, we refer to the combinations of the several foods, we find large numbers who disliked them. Thus acids were objected to by 29; sugar, 25.7; tea, 11.6; coffee, 17.3; vegetables, 2.1; fruits, 5; bread, 6.1; meat, 4.3; milk, 6.1; and fat by 66.6 per cent. Acids and fat were alone objected to by 10; acids, sugar, and fat alone by 3.2; sugar and fat alone by 5.4; coffee and fat, and tea and fat, each by .7 per cent.; and bread and fat alone by 1 per cent. The various other combinations amount to 66 in number, and offer much interest.

We further sought to ascertain if there were any differences in those cases in which the perspiration was usually free and in those who were commonly liable to have perspirations of an acid odour, and the following results were obtained:—

Of those who disliked acids, 36.6 per cent. were liable to much perspiration, 31.8 per cent. had acid, and 37.1 per cent. had not acid perspirations. Of those who disliked fat, 78.8 per cent. had much perspiration; in 69.2 per cent. the perspirations were acid, and in 58.5 per cent. there was no perception of the acidity. Of those who perspired with unusual readiness or to an unusual degree, 35.2 per cent. disliked sugar, 15.4 per cent. disliked tea, and 28.1 per cent. objected to coffee. Those who experienced acid perspirations and disliked tea, sugar, and coffee, were 37.3, 14.2, and 24.1 per cent.

There was a great similarity in these particulars to those obtained from persons in whom general asthenia was the leading feature, but great dissimilarity to those found in chronic bronchitis. Thus the dislike of fat with much perspiration was in phthisis, debility, and bronchitis, 78.8, 78.5, and 42.8 per cent., and the same dislike associated with acid perspirations was in the three diseases 69.2, 72.4, and 38.4 per cent. There was a larger proportion of cases of debility which disliked acids, with much perspiration and with sour perspirations, than in phthisis.

In reference to the dislike for sugar, tea, and coffee, there was not absolute uniformity in the results, as may be seen by the following table:—

TABLE No. 1.

Showing the Percentage of those who dislike Sugar, Tea, and Coffee, with certain Conditions of the Perspiration.

	Phthisis.	Debility.	Bronchitis.
Perspire much—			
Dislike Sugar	35.2	35.	41.
" Tea	15.4	7.	14.
" Coffee	28.1	14.	35.
Have Acid Perspiration—			
Dislike Sugar	37.3	30.	34.
" Tea	14.2	10.	15.
" Coffee	24.1	37.	21.5

The dislike for sugar was nearly equal in the three diseases. Tea was less frequently disliked by the cases of debility than by those of phthisis and bronchitis, whilst there was a want of uniformity in the taste for coffee.

We also instituted another special inquiry into the prevalence of a distaste for the various kinds of fat, and of meat and milk, and now proceed to quote the results.

DISTASTE FOR FAT.

The prevalence of a distaste for fat was determined by an inquiry made upon five hundred cases at the Hospital for Consumption, of persons suffering from phthisis in the several stages, bronchitis, debility, and derangement of the liver. The fats selected for inquiry were fat of meat, butter, suet, milk, and fat of bacon, and the results obtained are inserted in the following table :—

Table No. 2.

Showing the Frequency with which Fat Food, in various Combinations, is Eaten in Disease.

F signifies fat meat, B butter, S suet in puddings, Mk milk, and Ba fat bacon. The italics show that the fat was liked little, whilst the small capitals indicate that it was liked much.

Kind of Fat eaten.	In-patients, all Stages.	Phthisis.				Bronchitis.	Debility.	Liver, etc.
		All Stages.	Out-patients.					
			Destruction.	Consolidation.	Very Early.			
F B S Mk Ba	...	62	27	24	11	46	15	6
F B S Mk Ba	...	17	9	5	3	5	5	...
F B S Mk Ba	...	1	1	...	...	1	1	...
F *B* S Mk Ba	...	...	...	...	...	...	1	...
F B S Mk *Ba*	...	3	1	2	...	...	1	...
F *B* S Mk *Ba*	...	2	2	...	...	...	...	...
F n S Mk *Ba*	...	2	1	1	...	...	...	...
F B S Mk ʙᴀ	...	1	1	...	...	...	...	...
F B S Mk *Ba*	...	3	1	1	1	...	1	...
F B S Mk Ba	...	2	1	1	...	...	...	...
F ʙ S Mk ʙᴀ	...	1	1	...	...	...	...	...
F ʙ S Mk Ba	...	1	...	1	...	...	...	...
F B S Mk *Ba*	...	1	...	1	...	...	...	...
F B S ᴍᴋ Ba	...	1	...	1	...	...	...	...
F B S ᴍᴋ *Ba*	...	1	...	...	1	...	...	...
F B S Mk *Ba*	...	1	...	...	1	...	...	...
F B S Ba	1	2	1	...	1	...	...	...
F B S Mk	52	12	4	6	2	3	1	1
F B S Mk	1	...	...	...	...	...	...	...
Carry forward								

TABLE No. 2—*continued.*

Kind of Fat eaten.	In-patients, all Stages.	Phthisis. All Stages.	Out-patients. Destruction.	Consolidation.	Very Early.	Bronchitis.	Debility.	Liver, etc.
Brought forward								
F B S Mk	...	...	...	...	...	...	1	...
F B S Mk	1	2	2	...	...	...	...	...
F B S Mk	18	8	3	3	2	1	1	...
F B S	1	...	...	...	...	...	...	...
F B S	1	...	...	...	...	...	...	...
F B S	1	...	...	...	...	...	...	...
F Mk	...	1	...	1	...	...	...	...
F D Mk	1	...	...	...	...	...	...	...
F B Mk	1	...	...	...	...	...	...	...
F D Mk	...	...	...	...	...	...	1	...
F S *Mk*	...	...	...	...	...	...	1	...
F S Mk Ba	...	...	...	...	...	1	...	...
F S Mk *Ba*	...	1	...	...	1	...	...	...
F S	...	...	...	...	...	...	1	...
B S Mk Ba	1	7	5	1	1	1	1	...
B S мк Ba	...	1	1	...	...	...	...	...
B S Mk Ba	1	17	9	4	4	5	2	3
B S Mk *Ba*	...	4	1	2	1	1	...	...
B S Mk Ba	...	1	1	...	...	...	...	...
B S Mk *Ba*	...	2	1	...	1	...	1	...
B S Mk Ba	...	2	...	2	...	...	1	...
B S Mk BA	...	1	...	1	...	...	1	...
B S Mk *Ba*	...	...	...	...	...	...	1	...
B S Mk	34	23	12	7	4	2	7	6
B S *Mk*	...	1	1	...	...	...	...	...
B S *Mk*	...	2	1	...	1	...	1	...
B S Mk	...	2	1	...	1	1	2	...
B S мк	1	1	1	...	...	...	1	...
B S Mk	...	3	...	2	1	...	...	...
B S Mk	...	2	...	1	1	1	...	1
B Mk Ba	...	1	1	...	...	...	...	...
B Mk Ba	...	2	...	1	1	...	1	...
B Mk	...	2	2	...	...	...	...	...
B Mk	12	3	1	...	2	...	1	1
B *Mk*	1	2	...	1	1	1	1	...
B S	1	1	...	1	...	1	...	...
B S	1	...	...	...	...	...	...	...
B	3	1	1	...	...	...	...	...
S Mk Ba	...	1	1	...	...	...	...	...
S Mk *Ba*	...	1	1	...	...	...	...	...
S Mk *Ba*	...	...	...	...	...	1	...	...
S Mk	1	2	2	...	...	1	...	...
Mk Ba	...	1	...	...	1	...	...	...
Mk	3	3	2	1	...	...	1	...
Total number examined	137	213	99	71	45	72	51	18

TABLE No. 3.

Showing the Percentage of the Cases in which the various Fats were taken in Disease.

Kind of Fat eaten.	In-patients, all Stages.	Phthisis.				Bronchitis.	Debility.	Liver, etc.
		All Stages.	Out-patients.					
			3d.	2d.	1st.			
Fat	56.1	58.3	55.5	65.2	53.5	79.1	58.8	83.3
Bacon . . .	...	66 8	76.6	66.6	65.1	84.7	60.7	50.
Suet	83.5	93.3	94.	95.6	88.	98.6	64.7	95.
Butter . . .	94.2	95.7	95.	97.1	95.3	95.8	94.1	100.
Milk	92.8	98.1	98.	98.5	97.6	97.2	98.	100.
5 Elements . .	...	46.4	...	...	...	72.2	47.	38.8
4 " . .	...	28.4	...	...	...	16.6	1.7	16 6
3 " . .	...	18.0	...	...	...	.7	2.7	38.8
2 " . .	...	.52	...	...	...	...	...	.55
1 " . .	...	.19	...	...	...	...	...	

Of the 213 phthisical out-patients, 46 per cent. ate all the kinds of fat; 28 per cent. ate four kinds; 18 per cent. ate three kinds; $\frac{1}{2}$ of 1 per cent. ate only two kinds; and not $\frac{2}{10}$ of 1 per cent. were limited to one kind only. By way of parenthesis, we may state, that if milk be regarded as one of the fats, only three patients ate milk exclusively, and hence some of the other fats were taken by 210 of 213 cases. The number of cases by which each of the fats was taken, was in the out-patients as follows: Fat meat was taken by 58 per cent.; bacon fat, 66 per cent.; suet, 93 per cent.; butter, 95 per cent.; and milk, 98 per cent. The quantities are in each case a little higher than those obtained from the in-patients; but we rely upon them, since the in-patients, being asked the question in parties, were somewhat influenced in their answers each by the other, as shown by a tendency to uniformity in the answers of each party of patients; whereas the out-patients were asked singly. It is also quite possible, that their tastes may have been slightly changed during their residence in the hospital, and thus fewer persons liking suet may be owing to the surfeit which some of them get with the milk and suet supper.

We have inserted the results obtained from other conditions than those under discussion, both from their own interest, and as facts with which those observed in the early stages of phthisis may be compared. The highly important fact was elicited that fat is less commonly liked in phthisis than in other diseased conditions of the system, and that this dislike is more general in persons afflicted with the disease in its early than in those suffering from the subsequent stages of the disease. Thus, 58.3 per cent. of those in all

stages of phthisis liked some form of fat, but in the early stage
alone the number was reduced to 53.5 per cent., so that nearly half
of all cases of early phthisis have a distaste for fat. In reference
to the kind of fat which was most disliked at this early period, we
remark that only 37.7 per cent. liked all the kinds of fat; 28.8 per
cent. disliked fat bacon; .23 per cent. disliked milk; 6.6 per cent.
disliked butter; 44.4 per cent. disliked fat of meat; and 9 per cent.
disliked suet in puddings.

DISTASTE FOR MEAT AND MILK.

The diminution in the relish for meat is much less than that for
fat, but it is more evident in the early than in the advanced conditions of the disease. In this particular there is doubtless much
diversity, but it will commonly be found that in the conditions in
which there is any material diminution of appetite, the distaste for
meat is greater than for other prime articles of food. In the advanced conditions, there is still a tolerable and in some cases a good
appetite for flesh meat. In an inquiry in which we noted all the
ingesta and egesta of fifteen phthisical cases for a month in the
summer season, it was found that the average quantity of cooked
mutton without bone which the several cases ate was as follows, in
ounces: 3.7, 3.6, 3, 3.6, 5.9, 4.6, 5.4, 5.4, 5.4, 6, 6.9, and 4.5,
or a total average quantity of 4.83 ounces. In all these instances
the supply of meat was unlimited, and as they were all men, and
belonged to the working classes, it must be admitted that whilst the
quantity taken was considerable, it was below that which healthy
men similarly situated would have eaten.

The diminution in the relish for milk is ordinarily not very great,
and when there is a distaste for that article of food, it is frequently
found that it had existed in a state of health. The foregoing table
(No. 3) shows in how few cases there was an entire dislike to milk
in this early stage of the disease; but when large numbers of cases
are considered, we believe that a dislike has been acquired much
more commonly than the table indicates. It is, however, to be observed, that when a dislike occurs, it is almost always based upon a
belief that the milk does not agree with the system, and that it
scarcely ever occurs that there is any true dislike to milk when
made into puddings.

DIGESTION.

*There is commonly some derangement of the function of digestion,
but it is frequently small, and in such cases is not important.*

The evidences which we would adduce in support of this proposition are that the tongue is more or less discoloured, or loaded with
a buff-coloured coat, and presents enlarged and projecting papillæ,
and is not unfrequently large and flabby. Also that there is a

sense of oppression after meals, and tenderness over the epigastrium on pressure, at most periods of the day; a sour taste in the mouth, and flatulency. These conditions are more commonly found with the lymphatic temperament, whilst in many of the sanguineo-nervous temperament the tongue retains its usual size and colour, and remains clean. It is very frequent in dressmakers, tailors, shoemakers, and others of sedentary occupations; in printers and others living in foul air, and engaged in night work; and in the poor, who live chiefly upon bread, potatoes, and tea; and in all such instances it is a prominent symptom, and demands prime attention. In a majority of such cases there is much intolerance of fat, and occasionally we have met with instances in which fat caused pain at the stomach.

AMOUNT OF FOOD TAKEN.

The amount of food taken is commonly somewhat lessened.

In the inquiry referred to at page 51 it was found that in the various stages of phthisis combined, there was a diminution in the total quantity of solid food consumed. The quantity taken by the several cases in ounces was as follows, on the average of a month in May and June: 18.9, 19.5, 18.7, 26.4, 24.7, 26.9, 28.8, 21.4, 22.1, 31, 32.2, 41.5, and 22, or a total average of 25.5 ounces. The average amount of solids eaten in health, as deduced from our own inquiries, is from thirty-five to forty ounces, and hence it is manifest that, notwithstanding the existence of a tolerable appetite for food, there was a considerable diminution in the total weight of food taken. We have reason to believe that there is the same proportionate diminution in the food taken in the early stage, at least in the majority of cases—a diminution beyond that which the patient is aware of, until closely questioned upon the subject.

ASSIMILATION.

The assimilation of food is commonly defective.

The degree of assimilation of food is chiefly to be proved by the weight and general condition of the system, and as we shall show that they are usually reduced whilst there is a moderate quantity of food taken, it will follow that there is less assimilation of nutritive material. This fact is capable of determination in a more exact way, by ascertaining the proportion of the elements of a given quantity of food which remains in the bowel as compared with that which occurs in health, for we have proved by our experiments in prisons[1] that, under conditions in which there was lessened assimilation of food, there was an unusual quantity of nitrogenous matter remaining in the bowel, and which consequently had not entered the blood. We hope to find opportunity to determine this fact experimentally

[1] Phil. Trans. 1861.

in phthisis. In the absence of these inquiries we must fall back upon the external evidences of mal-assimilation, and shall be able to show that the general system is not well nourished.

WEIGHT AND BULK OF THE BODY.

The weight and bulk of the body are almost universally lessened.
We believe this proposition to be true in the great majority of instances, and when it appears to be otherwise we would counsel a careful inquiry into the facts at all the periods of the disease. It is quite true that cases of isolated tuberculous masses have been found after death, which were unconnected with any known change of health during life, but that is not satisfactory evidence—and we know of instances in which there are the evidences of deposition, and yet the person remains in apparently sound health ; but we contend that in almost all instances careful inquiry will show that at the period of origin of the disease there was loss of flesh and weight extending over some months. This diminution of weight and bulk is often only temporary, even in those cases in which the disease slowly progresses ; and either by the unassisted powers of nature acting in the cycle of the seasons, or by more careful attention to hygienic conditions, it passes away for a time, and the weight again becomes nearly normal. So general, however, is this loss of weight, that we should expect to find it in every case.
But the fact being admitted, it is necessary to consider what importance should be attached to it. As ordinarily understood, it is referred to the solid structures of the body, and to the muscular or nitrogenous tissues in particular, and hence great importance is commonly attached to this sign as an evidence of defective nutrition. Upon this point recent experimental inquiries have thrown much light, and we will endeavour in a few words to explain the position of this question at the present moment.
The weight of the body depends upon the amount of food and excretions contained within the body, of the fluids in the circulation and in the tissues, of the more solid parts of the soft tissues, and lastly of the heavy and comparatively unchangeable bones. Hence, variation in any of these numerous sources will influence the total weight of the body.
The errors due to the food and excretions may be almost removed by taking the weight of the body before breakfast, and after feces and urine have been passed ; but this cannot be effected at any other period of the day.
The variations in the amount of fluid in the body which occur under normal conditions are exceedingly great, and refer to the water contained both in the blood and in the tissues. It is evident that there will be more fluid in the blood within an hour and a half after a meal than will be found immediately before the following

meal. We have also shown elsewhere[1] that as the excretion of
fluid is lessened in the latter part of the day, there must be an increase in the quantity of blood at that period; and this in our own
case is so constant and to such a degree, that we usually weigh from
one pound and a half to two pounds more at 11 P. M. than at 8
A. M. We have also shown that the excretion of fluid is materially
influenced by temperature and barometric pressure, when acting
suddenly; so that increased atmospheric pressure induces increased
elimination of urine on the same day, and increased temperature
the contrary effect, either on the same or following day. With a
falling thermometer and a rising barometer, as in frosty weather,
there is great increase in the elimination, whilst with a rising thermometer and a rising barometer the effect is scarcely perceptible,
since in the former case two co-ordinate actions reinforce each other,
whilst in the latter two opposed actions neutralize each other.
Hence variations of meteorological conditions exert great influence
upon the body, and vary its weight greatly, so that it increases
in the summer and diminishes in the winter. Moreover, whenever
from any cause there is a large elimination of urine, there will be
on the following days, or there was on the preceding day, a corresponding diminution, as the following examples in health prove :—

Alternations		$\left\{\begin{array}{l}\text{64, 40, 71, 44, 66, and 83 fl. oz.}\\ \text{57, 37, 62, 44, 60, and 46 fl. oz.}\end{array}\right.$
Waves	. . .	73, 50, 41, 41, 57, 52, 54, and 63 fl. oz.
Increase	. . .	44, 38, 60, 62, and 74 fl. oz.
Decrease	. . .	68, 49, 49, 40, 42, 37, and 26 fl. oz.

Hence, whilst these variations in a long period neutralize each other,
and thus tend to keep the body of uniform weight, they disturb the
weight in each direction when regarded for short periods.

The elimination of fluid is also influenced greatly by the quantity
of fluid ingested, by the kind of food, and by exertion. Thus, a
quantity of fluid taken upon an empty stomach before breakfast,
causes the emission of about thrice its own weight within three hours;
but if food be taken, the emission is greatly reduced, and a large
portion of the water becomes fixed in the body. In the latter case
the food prevented both the emission of the water which had been
drunk, and the further quantity which would have been otherwise
educed by the fluid taken. With much food, much water is fixed,
and *vice versâ;* and hence, when the appetite is lessened and food
is diminished, the emission of fluid is thereby increased.

In reference to kind of food, we believe ourselves justified in stating that fat, flesh, and animal foods have the greatest power to
prevent the elimination of fluids; whilst, on the other hand, starchy
food allows the elimination. This is observed in practice; for those
who live well on animal food often retain a larger bulk than the ill
fed. Hence, when the appetite for fat and flesh is lessened, there

will be an increase in the elimination of fluid, and the weight of the body will be thereby decreased.

We have also proved that when in ordinary conditions of health there has been a day of comparative fasting from both fluids and solids, there was much less elimination of fluid on the following day, when the usual quantity of fluid and solid food was eaten, than would have occurred under normal conditions.

Rest preceded by exertion always tends to prevent elimination of fluid on the day of rest, upon the principle which was active in all these researches, viz., that during the period of exertion there was an unusual emission of fluid, and during the subsequent rest nature restored the balance by temporarily fixing a larger quantity of fluid.

We need not stay to prove that a variation in the quantity of fat in the body will cause a considerable variation in the weight, and have only to remark, that this applies not only to the fat deposited in the skin, but to that in muscle, to the extent of fifty per cent., if we may quote experiments made upon well-fed animals. We believe that so long as fat is abundantly supplied from without and duly assimilated, or there is an excess of fat in the body which may be consumed, so long is there a power to withhold the extreme emission of fluids; and therefore, when a person is losing fat, he not only loses weight *pari passu* with the loss of fat, but when the store of fat is exhausted, he loses weight in a rapidly-increasing ratio from the more rapid elimination of fluid, until that bulk and weight are attained which are consistent with the existing state of health and the kind and amount of food supplied. Thus, in the case of persons in training for violent exertion, or in that of prisoners on the tread-wheel, where the amount of animal food supplied is abundant, the weight lessens only as the fat and superfluous fluid disappear; but after no long time an arrest of this process occurs, and the muscles retain their bulk. In conditions in which there is not a sufficiency of animal food, or, as in the disease now under consideration, there is defective assimilation of food, the loss of weight continues after the fat has been removed. Hence it follows that loss of appetite for fat and flesh has far greater influence over the weight of the body than the loss of weight of these substances will account for.

We have now seen how many sources of loss of weight there are, without having any reference to the nitrogenous elements of the body. In reference to the muscular tissues, we must further observe that they consist of from twenty to fifty per cent. of fat, according to the condition of the body, and that in the lean of muscle alone there is about eighty per cent. of water. Every housewife knows how much more lamb will shrink in cooking than mutton, and the difference between a grass-fed and stall-fed ox is well seen in the greater loss of weight which the flesh undergoes in the process of roasting. We are also familiar with the fact that some flesh is soft, compressible, and flabby, whilst other is hard and resisting to the touch. All these prove that bulk and weight of flesh do not imply uniformity in nitrogenous elements, but are largely influenced by the fluids which are contained in the tissues. Hence, therefore, on the one hand, as by exertion, we may have an unusual emission of fluid from the muscles, and their weight and bulk be lessened with a relative increase of their nitrogenous elements, so on the other the weight and bulk of a muscle may be maintained whilst the nitrogenous elements are reduced and the contained water increased.

We have thus shown in how great a degree the components of the body may vary with change of weight and bulk; and it may well be asked if, with such diversity of cause, loss of weight in the early stage of phthisis means anything of general interpretation.

It follows that the diminution in weight and bulk which occurs in early phthisis is no necessary evidence of loss of nitrogenous tissue, much less that it is altogether explained by it. But when, as we have shown, there is some diminution in the food taken, when there is less perfect assimilation of food, and when fat is disliked, it will follow that the store of fat in the body will be lessened, that the elimination of fluid will be increased, that the nitrogenous parts of the body will be less perfectly restored, and that the tone of the tissues will be lowered. Hence, in such cases, loss of weight indicates numerous conditions of great importance.

CHAPTER VII.

ELIMINATION.

The fixation of fluid in the body is lessened, and the elimination of it increased.

We have already referred to this condition under the preceding heading, but shall now analyze it somewhat further.

We have shown the relation between the fixation and elimination of fluid on the one hand, and the quantity and kind of food on the other, and stated that there is lessened ingestion of fat and flesh, and a correspondingly larger elimination of water. The immediate result of this is to lessen the bulk of the body, and by diminishing the fulness of the tissues and the bloodvessels to give the sense of atonicity or flabbiness to the limbs. It also indicates, and is co-existent with lessened nutrition of the body. It is probable that this result is partly physical and partly vital, and commonly proceeds to a moderate degree only. It is also to be noted that whilst there is some diminution in the quantity of food, there is no diminution, but often an increase, in the quantity of fluid taken, and that this tends to increase the elimination of fluid.

We will now offer some remarks on the two principal eliminators of fluid, viz., the skin and the kidneys.

THE SKIN.

The action of the skin is commonly increased, either absolutely or relatively to the vital transformation.

In a majority of cases of early phthisis the skin is thin, fair, and very sensitive, and we believe it to be an indisputable fact, that at the early period of the disease as it is usually seen, apart from any evident inflammatory action, the skin is soft and cool and tends easily to perspire, and to this we attach the utmost importance.

The function of the skin is almost entirely that of the heat-regulator of the body, and in that capacity it rules almost every vital function. It is not, as is commonly supposed, an organ which, in case of need, may act vicariously for the lungs, for in our experiments, in which the whole body, except the head, was inclosed in a caoutchouc dress, through which a current of air was first passed, and then carried over a solution of potash, we only obtained six grains of carbonic acid per hour, or about 1.25 per cent. of that emitted by the lungs; and by similar experiments made on the Continent it has been proved that the quantity does not exceed 2 per cent. Hence it is manifest that, whatever may be the source of this carbonic acid, the quantity bears no such proportion to that which is emitted by the lungs, that the one organ can act vicariously for the other. Moreover, the structure of the two organs is so totally dissimilar that, *à priori*, it would be impossible to admit identity of function.

The skin acts as the heat-regulator of the body by radiating heat into and absorbing it from the atmosphere, and by the conversion of the fluid into vapour, which occurs upon its surface. We do not need to refer further to the two former processes, but shall offer some remarks upon the latter only.

It is well known that insensible evaporation or perspiration from the skin occurs at all times, and that, under favourable conditions, the quantity of fluid vapourized is so greatly increased, that being condensed in the air surrounding the body it becomes evident to the sight, or being condensed upon the body it rushes down the skin in streams. In this act of vaporization a large amount of heat is rendered latent, so that a given quantity of fluid being converted into vapour, the latter will require nearly one thousand times more latent heat than the former. The heat thus absorbed and rendered latent must be abstracted from the surrounding substances, and therefore chiefly from the skin upon which the process is proceeding. This explains the cooling effect of perspiration which all have noticed to follow exertion, or exposure to heat, or the ingestion of certain hot fluids, as tea, or the use of the hot air, vapour, or water bath.

It is chiefly by this means that uniformity of the temperature of the body is effected, under varying conditions. Thus after a meal, when vital actions are proceeding vigorously, and heat is being abundantly generated, the skin, as every other part of the body, becomes hot, and if this proceed to any great extent, and it be also dry, there is a sense of oppression induced, because the body cannot rid itself of its superfluous heat; but after the lapse of an hour or two, and especially after taking tea, the skin becomes soft and active, and vaporization cools the body. So when the vital actions are increased by exertion, and heat is abundantly generated, we know that the normal result is increased evaporation and perspiration; and the same explanation avails us to account for the power which the body has of keeping itself cooler than the surrounding air in the burning regions of the East. For these purposes it is necessary that the skin be in a condition in which evaporation may proceed, and that the circulation supply a sufficiency of fluid to the skin to meet this constant drain.

In the contrary condition of cold, the skin becomes less active and is dry, so that evaporation is reduced to a minimum, and the refrigeration of the body depends mainly upon radiation, and is regulated chiefly by clothing.

Hence it follows that the skin is almost omnipotent in preventing excess of heat, and acts as a self-regulator quite apart from our care, but it is almost powerless against the effect of cold, and we are then left to our discretion in protecting the body by clothing and shelter.

In the cases now under consideration this beneficial action of the skin is converted into an evil by being in excess of the requirements of the system, and its tendency is to cause too free elimination of the fluid from the body, to unduly reduce the temperature of the body, to injuriously interfere with the force of the heart's action, as we shall have hereafter more particularly to point out, and lastly and most importantly to waste the body by demanding an excess of vital transformation in order to maintain a supply of heat from within—a demand which cannot be supplied. Hence we have an explanation of the ill health and of the occurrence of phthisis in persons who exchange a hot for a much colder climate.

The amount of fluid which is thus lost by the skin may be approximately ascertained by the series of experiments which we made upon fifteen phthisical patients in May and June (already referred to at page 52).

The table No. 4, page 59, contains a number of facts to which we may hereafter have occasion to refer to supply the information which we now seek.

The part of this table to which we wish now to refer has reference to the relation of the egesta to the ingesta.

In the various cases referred to, the total fluid and solid egesta varied daily from 65.3 oz. to 143.1 oz., with an average extending over the month of 92.7 oz. The weight of the feces, sputa, and urine varied in the different cases from 29.7 oz. to 67.7 oz. or a

TABLE No. 4.

Showing the Daily Average Returns obtained from each and all of Fifteen Phthisical Patients, who were under observation during One Month; the weights in Avoirdupois ounces.

CASE	69	95	107	88	79	75	46	80	51	90	59	73	85	77	Total Average
Ingesta—Solid food	40.1	32.3	21.1	22.3	30.1	21.6	26.6	28.8	14.7	21.7	31.4	15.2	19.7	19.	24.8
" Fluid	103.	72.2	83.3	53.	63.3	60.	67.	62.6	92.8	43.6	82.6	62.	54.8	51.3	67.9
Total	143.1	105.5	101.4	75.2	93.4	81.6	93.6	91.2	107.5	65.3	114.	77.2	74.5	70.3	92.7
Egesta—Feces	7.	7.5	7.8	2.41	9.6	5.65	5.21	4.75	5.85	6.14	7.55	2.6	4.82	2.34	6.3
" Vomits			1.82		.20										.14
" Sputa and Saliva in Smoking	22.2	1.66	1.7	2.8	3.14	.77	5.	1.9	.75	5.2	2.2	6.9	2.	1.73	2.8
" Urine	58.5	36.8	50.8	36.2	32.2	42.5	39.8	32.6	64.	21.	49.5	23.9	30.	25.7	38.8
Total	67.7	55.6	62.1	41.4	45.1	48.9	50.	39.25	70.6	32.3	59.5	32.4	36.5	29.7	48.04
Excess of Ingesta over Egesta	75.3	49.5	42.2	33.8	48.2	32.6	43.6	52.95	36.9	33.	64.4	44.8	38.	40.5	44.66
Weight of body	+2.8	+.1	+1.4	+.6	+2.1	+1.1	-.4	+.7	=	+.1	+2.2	+.8	-2.2	+.4	+.6
Solids in urine (grains)	1226	856	776	758	732	704	676	626	604	596	592	574	574	550	703
Pulsation	84.1	86.4	92.6	91.3	92.7	83.2	96.9	94.4	76.1	97.5	89.3	104.6	128.4	112.5	95.3
Respiration	16.	22.6	24.9	18.	20.6	17.	22.7	20.6	22.4	24.7	25.6	31.	20.6	29.7	23.
Meat and Fish	6.8	6.2	5.2	5.4	4.1	4.3	•3.8	4.7	.5	4.2	5.2	3.1	3.7	4.	4.4
Wine			2.6		.8					1.1		1.4		.9	.5
Ale and Porter	15.1	8.2	14.7	19.	8.7	8.	10.	7.4	8.	2.4	8.	9.1	8.	10.	10.
Bread	21.7	18.4	9.1	8.7	14.	9.1	15.6	11.	6.8	8.6	16.6	8.4	7.1	8.2	12.

total average of 48.04 oz.   The excess of the ingesta over the egesta
varied from 32.6 oz. to 75.3 oz., with an average quantity of 44.66
oz., and if we deduct from that amount the carbon exhaled by the
lungs, nearly the whole remainder will represent the fluid which
passed off by the skin and lungs.   The amount of carbon evolved
was not ascertained, but from our inquiries upon persons in health
we find that 19½ grs. of carbon are expired daily in quietude to each
pound of body-weight, and as the average weight of these patients
was 135 lbs. the total daily elimination of carbon in health may be
estimated at 6 oz. daily, and in a state of disease at five-sixths of
that amount.   Hence the amount of vapour eliminated by the skin
and lungs was about 40 oz. per day, and this abstracted from the
body nearly 40,000 times as much heat as was held latent by that
quantity of fluid when within the body.

Hence in the class of cases now under consideration we find the
skin unusually active and abstracting heat rapidly from the body,
when, at the same time, there is less transformation of nutriment
than occurs in health, and consequently less heat produced within
the body.   As a necessary result the temperature of the body is
reduced, the hands and feet become cold, and the depression and
exhaustion of the nervous power ensues, which is known to occur
with excess of cold of the body.   In an inquiry made upon 1,000
phthisical patients, we found that 54 per cent. were *constitutionally*
liable to coldness of the extremities.   Of these 4.8 per cent. suffered
from coldness of the hands, and 19.1 per cent. from coldness of the
feet alone; whilst in 30.2 per cent. that condition affected both the
extremities in the same person.   This was observed in states of so-
called health, but it must be much in excess of the frequency occurring in robust constitutions.

URINE.

*The amount of urine evolved is perhaps equal to that in health,
but varies with the activity of other outlets of the body.*

We have shown in inquiries which were prosecuted upon ourself
throughout the year, that there is very great variation in the amount
of urine evolved in health at the different seasons of the year, and
also that there is a relation between the amount of fluid evolved
through this and other outlets.   The experiments in phthisical cases
just referred to, although extending over a long period, may not be
taken to represent the quantity of urine which would be evolved at
all seasons of the year, and must, therefore, be accepted with a certain amount of reservation.   Moreover, we have shown that in these
cases there was a very active state of the skin, and consequently a
large amount of fluid passed away from the body by that outlet,
and less would remain to be eliminated by the kidneys.   The daily
amount of urine varied from 21 oz. to 64 oz., and the average of all
fourteen cases was 38.8 oz. during the whole summer month.   The

amount of urine in health varies greatly in different persons, and it is very difficult to obtain a standard with which it would be just to compare any individual case, or a few cases, but it is probable that the average now obtained is not less than occurs in health.

SPECIFIC GRAVITY.

We do not purpose to enter into a consideration of the quality of the urine evolved in phthisis, but as an American observer[1] has made the unaccountable observation, that "in phthisis, as a general thing, its specific gravity does not exceed 1010," we think it right to cite the specific gravity in the cases of phthisis now referred to. The specific gravity was determined with great care, by means of an instrument with a large bulb, and graduated to a quarter of a degree, and at the same time the exact temperature of the urine was determined.

TABLE No. 5.

Showing the Specific Gravity + 1000 in the Day and Night Urine in Eight Cases of Phthisis daily during One Month.

CASE.	No. 90.		No. 93.		No. 95.		No. 88.		No. 79.		No. 75.		No. 73.	
	N.	D.	N.	D.	N.	D.	N.	D.	N.	D.	N.	D.	N.	D.
May 15	26.	30.	11.	14.	18.	28.	14.5	24	16.	30.3	17.	16.5	15.	30.
" 16	25.	28.	12.5		21.2	31.	21.5	26.2	16.8	31.	18.2	19.	25.	25.
" 17	21.	25.	12.	14.5	20.	27.3	18.5	24.	17.	29.	20.	12.	25.	26.
" 18	25.	27.	14.	16.	22.	28.3	22.	26.	18.	13.7	16.3	12.6	25.	23.6
" 19	26.6	28.5	14.8	17.5	15.	29.	9.	23.	18.5	29.5	15.	7.	27.5	
" 20	27.	26.5	16.5	15.5	31.	40.	26.	21.	25.5	31.	15.	13.8	27.5	25.
" 21	25.	27.	14.5	17.	28.	30.2	12.6	23.5	16.6	27.	10.5	10.	25.2	28.
" 22	22.7	29.5	12.0	13.8	26.3	30.5	18.3	21.	14.5	52.	17.	15.8	22.3	28.
" 23	25.8	28.2	14.8	20.4	25.	22.	22.	21.	17.5	27.	13.	11.8	25.5	26.
" 24	24.	28.5	13.	14.	12.	28.	14.7	21.8	25.8	29.	15.5	19 7	17.	18.5
" 25	16.8	25.5	11.	12.	25.	27.	15.	23.5	27.5	23.8	15.	22.5	0.6	26.
" 26	24.	27.5	10.7	11.	25.	28.	16.8	13.5	22.	27.	14.	19.3	15.2	26.
" 27	27.5	25.	9.	11.5	28.	29.5	20.8	23.	27.3	26.5	14 2	15.4	22.3	24.5
" 28	25.	25.3	11.	11 5	26.5	29.	18.8	24.0	24.	29.	18.	17.	24.5	28.5
" 29	24.	26.5	8.5	11.5	23.	29.	17.8	23.	28.	26.	No. 77.		25.	24.
" 30	26.5	28 6	9.5	11.	19.	27.5	16.8	22.	29.	37.	18.7	22.3	12.	25.5
" 31	24.8	25.	9.0	11.6	23.5	27.	17.	20.2	25.5	33.5	20.5	24.	12.2	26.5
June 1	21.	28.6	9.5	9.5	16.5	27.	21.5	16.	24.	26.8	25.	24.	21.5	27.5
" 2	26.	24.	8.	9.8	7.5	24.8	17.	25.	26.5	34.	18.6	22.0	23.	25.
" 3	25.5	25.			12.5	27.5	25.8	22.5	25.	24.5	18.6	22.5	20.3	23.5
" 4	25.2	28.			22.	29.	22.3	25.	12.9	27.	16.	24.	20.5	26.
" 5	17.8	25.			15.8	27.	17.5	10.6	14.	30.	15.5	20.5	22.4	24.
" 6	28.	23.5			17.8	31.8	12.5	19.7	14.8	27.8	10.	23.	22.	27.
" 7	25.8	28.			18.5	22.	18.5	24.6	16.6	25.7	20.3	24.	20.	25.
" 8	25.8	26.5			12.6	27.5	25.	19.	16.5	31.	20.5	23.5	24.	28.3
" 9	25.5	25.5			19.	28.	12.	18.6	22.	17.4	20.	26.5	25.	28.5
" 10	27.	21.5			20.	26.	20.	21.8	34.	32.	20.	23.	23 8	23.
" 11	24.	27.			17.8	26.2	11.5	21.	14.8	13.8	18.2	20.	21.6	25.2

[1] Extracted from the "Phil. Med. Reporter," Sept. 21, by "Dublin Med. Press," Nov. 13, 1861.

The inquiry was made in the day and night urine separately, and as the whole returns are too voluminous, we insert in the preceding table a copy of the record in the first eight cases.

It will be observed that there was much diversity in the returns of the specific gravity, so that on one occasion it was so low as 1007, and in several others as high as 1030. Usually that of the night urine (9 P.M. to 8 A.M.) was less than that of the day. We cannot determine the true average specific gravity in these cases without the laborious process of multiplying each return by the number of ounces of urine of the day and night separately, and adding the totals, but it will suffice if we represent the number of occasions on which certain specific gravities were found. Thus,

A specific gravity of 1030 and upwards was found in 4.3 per cent.
  "   1020 "   " 65.0 "
  "   less than 1010 " 2.4 "

and hence it is quite clear that the specific gravity was certainly not less than in health.

As we intend on a future occasion to analyze the returns of two large series of inquiries which we have made, into the chemical and other qualities of the urine in phthisis, we shall not enter more fully into this question on the present occasion.

PERSPIRATION.

Perspirations are common in the early, as in the latter stages of phthisis, and oftentimes have a sour odour.

Of 177 cases of phthisis we found 40.1 per cent. had *constitutionally* a tendency to perspire much, 46.7 per cent. perspired as is usual, and 27.3 per cent. were believed to perspire less than others in health. In cases of debility and bronchitis there was a somewhat greater tendency to perspire. In a comprehensive inquiry, including one thousand phthisical persons, we recorded that 25.4 per cent. had been ascertained to perspire with unusual freedom in health.

It is common to regard the occurrence of considerable perspiration as a mark of the advanced stage of the disease; but in this we think there is an error. It cannot be doubted that profuse perspirations occur in the exhaustion of the later stage, and more commonly than at any other period; but it is equally true that they are met with, in a less degree, in a majority of cases of the early stage. This may be inferred from the remarks already made (p. 57), but they occur in an intermitting manner, and chiefly in the evening and in the early morning, whilst the patient sleeps. They also are observed whenever the heat is suddenly increased, as also with the sudden occurrence of cold weather in the autumn, upon any unusual exertion, and on the occasion of sudden surprise. The cause of this occurrence is to be found in the preternatural action of the skin, and particularly with that low state of the vital powers, which we have shown to occur at night, both in health and in disease. We are unable to explain the precise mode by which the degree of activity of the skin is regulated; but in reference to the latter, we have ascertained the rate of pulsation and respiration, and the amount of carbonic acid evolved at each hour of the day and night, and have proved that the vital actions are reduced during the night to a point not higher than from one-half to two-thirds of that which is found during the day. Whether, therefore, a state of atonicity occurs in the night, which leads to the more rapid elimination of fluid by the skin, we perhaps cannot prove, but the correlation of the two facts quite corresponds with other observations both in health and disease, viz., that with debility, or a diminished degree of vital power, there is commonly increased tendency to perspire. We have also noticed that perspirations occur in feeble persons who sleep when lying upon the back, and in whom the tongue, falling back into the pharynx, induces increased dyspnœa. In such instances the patient sleeps uneasily, and wakes bathed in perspiration; but on awaking, the respirations become more natural, and the perspirations gradually cease.

We have also observed two conditions of the perspiration which must have a significance both in reference to the condition of the system and as an indication for treatment. Normally, the perspiration is slightly acid—a condition due, we believe, not to secondary changes, as some chemists are inclined to think, but to the fixed and volatile acids which have been detected in that fluid. The amount of acid varies at different periods of the day, so that before breakfast it is the least, and if much exertion be then made, it will be found that the perspiration is perfectly neutral, whilst after meals, and particularly in the afternoon, the degree of acidity is increased. We have noticed that in numerous cases of phthisis the acidity of the perspiration is so increased that the odour has attracted the attention of the patient, and particularly in the more marked perspirations which occur in the early morning. In some it is so pungent as to be perceptible, and sometimes very offensive, in every part of the room, whilst in other cases there is no acid odour, however profuse may be the perspiration. In the former case, we have constantly taken pains to prove that it occurs in cleanly persons, and after daily washing of the whole body, and when using clean linen, and is therefore not resulting from the circumstances too commonly found in the working classes. Of 177 cases of phthisis, 56.4 per cent. had a constitutional tendency to acid perspirations; whilst of those who perspired much, 70.7 per cent. had sour perspiration, and of those who perspired less than usual, 54.2 per cent. had remarked the acidity of the excretion. Hence phthisical persons appear to be constitutionally predisposed to an acid state of the perspiration.

We do not attempt any sufficient explanation of these conditions, but that which most readily occurs is the deficiency of alkali in the blood, whereby the final transformation into carbonic acid is prevented, and which must lead to, as it would be indicative of, lessened respiratory changes. We shall subsequently show that this inference is to a great extent supported by the effect of treatment. In many of these cases the linen is stained of a yellow colour, after having been worn but a day or two. The impression has been conveyed to our mind that in the cases in which there is considerable perspiration without any acid odour, there is very marked debility of system.

CHAPTER VIII.

TEMPERATURE OF THE BODY.

There is a general tendency to defect of temperature of the body.

We have already referred to this subject in Chapters VI. and VII. The temperature of the body bears a relation to the formation and supply of heat on the one hand, and the dispersion of heat on the other.

In reference to the supply of heat we have already shown that those vital processes upon which the production of heat within the body is dependent are in a greater or less degree lessened. With lessened transformation of food and lessened nutrition of the body there is diminished production of heat. In this climate, where the temperature of the external air is at all times below that of the body, there can be no gain of heat from without, since the loss will exceed the supply; but, on the contrary, there will be a loss, and particularly at the seasons of the year when the temperature is low and the air damp. In hot countries, however, the temperature of the external air approaches to or exceeds that of the body, and therefore there may be an abundant, nay, even an excessive supply from without which shall make good any defect in the production of heat within, and hence the condition now under consideration is far less powerful in hot than in cold climates, and in hot than in cold seasons. But in this country, if there be defect in the production of heat within, there must be absolute defect in the whole supply. The dispersion of heat chiefly depends upon the action of the skin and the protection of the body by clothing and shelter. It is quite evident that as there is a relation between the supply and the dispersion of heat, if the dispersion could be lessened in a degree commensurate with the diminution in the supply, the effect upon the system would be the same, so long as the total diminution was not so great as to act injuriously upon the system; but we have already shown that not only is there a lessened supply of heat but there is no diminution in the dispersion of it; nay, it often happens that there is both lessened supply and greater dispersion proceeding at the same time, and a marked total defect must follow. The action of the skin is, no doubt, the root of this evil, and is not under the control of the untaught individual, but there is an important subsidiary element, viz., the clothing of the body, which is within the control of those who may be able to obtain it. Of the former we will not now say more ; but, in reference to the latter, it is notorious how ill clad are many, both of the poor and rich, and how passively they submit to coldness of the hands, feet, and other uncovered parts from day to day.

These conditions are more frequently found in the young, in whom there is naturally great activity of the skin, and to whom activity of the vital functions is relatively of greater importance than at other periods of life.

The importance of this condition is both demonstrative and inferential. There can be no doubt that the maintenance of a certain degree of temperature is essential to the due performance of the vital actions, as is well seen in those who suffer from long exposure to cold. The long continuance of cold, moreover, reacts upon the body, and tends further to lessen the frequency of the circulation and the activity of the vital processes, and thus, in the conditions under consideration, it exerts a most injurious influence.

The occurrence of coldness of the hands and feet, and a general tendency to defect of heat, must at least imply that there is an inadequate supply of heat to the body, and should lead us to infer that the processes of nutrition are insufficiently performed, for, in the conditions in which we live, to be ill nourished is to be cold, and a continuance of these states must lead to deficient growth, and a depression of all the vital powers, inimical to health and dangerous to life (p. 60).

CHAPTER IX.

MUSCULAR POWER.

The muscular power is commonly lessened.

It is not at all times easy to prove this proposition, whilst in other cases the truth of it is very manifest. Many, especially the young. mistake will for power and ambition for capability, and with the moderate exertion made by females in the middle classes, it may often seem that the capability for walking and other ordinary modes of exertion remains unchanged. But in all cases there is an earlier sense of fatigue than occurs in health, and this is especially seen if there be unusual or somewhat laborious exertion, as going up hill or carrying weights. The muscles have also lost something of their tone, and feel less resisting on pressure. The thinner layers of the

4

muscles become relaxed, and dependent parts seem to hang more loosely. The pupil is not uncommonly enlarged, so as to give a bright and somewhat staring appearance to the eyes, and the muscles of the face do not so completely respond to the stimulus as to give full contractility and expression to the features. The eye kindles and the lips smile whilst there is vivacity of spirit, but there is a languor imprinted upon the features by the absence of the due contraction of the muscles of the face.

Such, indeed, must be the case if what has already been advanced have previously existed, for it is impossible that there should be full muscular tone and power with defective nutrition, innervation, and nitrogenous food, and with a tendency to defect in the temperature of the body. The condition of the muscular system is the sum of the conditions of health, just as the muscular system itself is the sum of the vital powers in a body, the essential feature of which is action and capability of motion. The least reflection shows that the muscular system is in truth *the body*, for the bones simply offer points of attachment and resistance to the levers, and the vital organs are employed in supplying it with food, and removing effete matters. The muscles are the end of the system, whilst the lungs and other organs are means to the end. Hence it follows that the condition of the muscular system is the true measure of the vital state of the system, and it cannot be perfect if any essential parts of the vital actions are imperfect.

CHAPTER X.

THE CIRCULATION.

The circulation is commonly enfeebled, and somewhat quickened.

We are accustomed to regard the circulation in two aspects, viz., the force and the rapidity of the current.

The force of the circulation is clearly dependent upon two conditions, viz., the *vis à tergo* and the *vis à fronte*. The propulsion of the current is due to the *vis à tergo* and the *vis insita*, if the latter exist; and if they be lessened, the force is lessened until it ceases. When fluid is impelled through smooth and partially-filled channels, there is but little resistance to the current, and the flow will be gentle and easy. As the channel becomes fuller, so the resistance is increased, assuming in all cases that the walls of the channel are not extensible; and in proportion as there is pressure made upon the walls, so will the resistance be further increased. If, with increasing resistance, there is no increase in the propelling power, the force of the current will become less; and, on the other hand, if the resistance be uniform, and the propelling power be increased, the impulse will be stronger. Hence, with much pressure, or *vis à fronte*, there must be much propulsion from the *vis à tergo*, and the greater the *vis à fronte*, the greater must be the *vis à tergo*, in order to maintain the circulation. Upon these principles we show the cause of the feeble circulation in early phthisis, and its importance upon the whole phenomena of nutrition.

If, as we have seen, the power of the muscular system be reduced and innervation be lessened, it follows that the *vis à tergo* of the heart upon the circulation is diminished also ; and if, as is believed, the *vis à tergo* which maintains the circulation in the veins be the action of the surrounding muscles, it again follows that the *vis à tergo* is lessened. On the other hand, if the various outlets of the capillaries be so increased in action that the contents of the bloodvessels pass through with unusual readiness, it follows that the *vis à fronte* is lessened. If the *vis à tergo* were lessened, the pulse must become softer ; how much more, then, when both the propulsion and the resistance are lessened ?

This argument, we believe, to apply to all cases in which there is rapid discharge of water from the blood, as in the case of dropsical effusions, great emission of urine, or perspiration ; but it is particularly applicable to the case of the active skin, with its immense network of capillaries, and its special apparatus for the elimination of water. With a soft and active skin, and a normal power of the heart, there must be a soft pulse ; then, how much more so when there is a soft and active skin, a feeble heart, and a feeble muscular power to maintain the venous current. Hence there is a chain of events, all of which hang together, and are amenable to one prime condition.

The importance of this condition, in reference to nutrition, is very evident. That a certain fulness of the capillaries generally is necessary to good nutrition may be inferred from the facts that vital actions are the most powerful after meals, when the bloodvessels are normally in their highest state of repletion, and lessen as the repletion lessens : and also that vigorous vital action, or nutrition, is not found with a feeble circulation and soft pulse. Hence we infer that in this condition there is not robust nutrition, whether the cause of it be primarily in defective nutrition of those structures upon the action of which the force of the circulation is dependent, or upon the diminution of the *vis à fronte*, or upon both conjoined.

We affirm, therefore, that in the early stage of phthisis a somewhat enfeebled circulation and soft pulse must be associated with the other conditions to which we have referred.

The rapidity of the circulation varies under every act which can affect the organism, and particularly with exertion and food. As we have fully discussed this elsewhere,[1] we will not here refer to it

[1] Health and Disease, as influenced by the daily, seasonal, and other Cyclical Changes in the Human System. (Walton & Maberly.)

further than to state that a meal will increase pulsation 15 to 30 beats per minute, that exertion will increase it from 15 to 130 per minute, according as we carry the body, at the rate of 1 mile to 8 miles per hour; that sleep in the daytime will lower the pulse 10 per minute, and in the night, with the other conditions of the night, will lower it to the further extent of 10 beats; and that ordinary idle rest will lower the pulse throughout the day to a considerable extent. It has been regarded as an established rule, that a rapid pulse indicates waste, and, if rapid beyond the normal standard, that it indicates debility. In the early stage of phthisis, the pulse is commonly either not quickened, or it is quickened in a moderate degree only; and there are cases in which it is, on the one hand slower, and on the other greatly quickened.

In the inquiry to which reference has already been made, in which the rate of pulsation was determined in each of the three postures of lying, sitting, and standing, at two periods of the day, viz., 8 A.M., before breakfast, and 4 P.M., before tea, on the large average of fifteen hundred observations in one month,[1] it was found that the average rate of pulsation in the different cases varied from 73 to 125 per minute in the morning, and from 79 to 131 in the evening, as shown in Table No. 6, p. 69.

Of these 15 cases in different stages of phthisis, one had a morning pulsation under 80, and 9 under 90 per minute; a rate beyond, but not greatly beyond, that of health; but in numerous instances in the early stage, and particularly in those of the lymphatic temperament, we have found a rate of pulsation below that of health.

What, then, is the significance of this fact? If there be unusually free elimination of fluid from the blood by any outlet, as, for example, the skin, and thereby the volume of the blood be reduced and the force of the circulation lessened, it is evident that, in order to maintain a due amount of vital action in the tissues of the body, the blood must be more rapidly distributed to them, or otherwise they cannot receive a due supply of that fluid. So, on the other hand, when the supply of blood is not thus interfered with, but is abundant, the rapidity of the circulation must be lessened, or the supply would become excessive. Hence feebleness and rapidity of pulsation are as naturally associated as are a full and slow pulse, and to alter the rapidity, if that were desirable, we must begin by changing the force. What, then, must be the condition in which a feeble and slow pulse is found? If a rapid and feeble pulse be indication of debility, how much more a slow and feeble pulse? And hence it is scarcely possible to attach too much importance to the latter as indicative of a system depressed and difficult to elevate.

The normal condition of the circulation in early phthisis is a certain amount of feebleness, with some increase in the rapidity, and so long as the rapidity is not very great, the conditions are as

[1] Bri. and For. Med.-Chir. Review, April, 1856.

Table No. 6.

Showing the Rate of Pulsation in Phthisis.

Æt.	22	34	45	18	20	31	?	Total Average	35	23	51	22	21	25	29	73
Average pulsation Morning, 8 A.M.	96.6	90.2	85.2	105.6	89.4	85.7	99.8	91.2	89.2	125.	73.1	89.8	97.1	80.8	82.1	87.1
Evening, 4 P.M.	110.3	103.7	97.3	118.4	100.4	93.5	103.6	98.4	96.	131.6	79.	95.6	102.5	85.7	85.6	85.6
Evening excess	13.7	13.5	12.1	11.8	11.	7.8	7.6	7.2	6.8	6.6	5.9	5.8	5.4	4.9	3.5	-1.5

Table No. 8.

Rate of Respiration in Phthisis.

Case, No.	73	77	93	68	107	90	46	51	95	79	80	83	88	73	69
Average rate	31.	28.7	27.3	25.6	24.9	24.7	22.7	20.4	22.6	20.6	20.6	20.6	18.1	17.	16.
Age, years	22	18	?	31	35	21	34	51	43	22	20	23	45	25	26

Table No. 9.

Order of Fifteen Cases of Phthisis in the Frequency of Respiration and Pulsation.

Respiration, Case No.	73	77	93	58	{80, 107}	{51, 46, 95}	{85, 80, 79}	75	69	95	83	69	75	51
Pulsation, Case No.	85	77	73	93	90	46	80	88	{107, 73}	58	88	95	69	51

favourable as they could be when allied with the disease. This is due both to lessened *vis à tergo* and *vis à fronte*, and the latter chiefly in connection with the skin.

Hence we do not consider that in early phthisis a moderate rapidity of circulation indicates an increase of vital action, whether destructive or otherwise, and, therefore, does not cause, nor does it show increased waste ; but, doubtless, there are cases in which there is marked rapidity of the circulation, which indicates increased vital changes of an inflammatory nature, but these are exceptional ones, and have a condition superadded to the phthisis. So there are many instances in highly sensitive young females, of sanguineo-nervous temperament, in whom there is almost perpetually increased rapidity of the circulation, due to emotional and similar influences, which must cause, and be indicative of, increased waste ; but however numerous these may be, they also must be classed apart from ordinary cases. The large mass of cases do not present either of these two conditions, when they are in their ordinary state, and examined under proper conditions.

CHAPTER XI.

RESPIRATION.

The respiration is shorter, shallower, feebler, and perhaps quicker.

When first questioned it commonly occurs that the patient is unaware of any shortness of breathing; but he subsequently admits that on any unusual exertion, as ascending stairs or running, his breath is short. He also frequently finds that this state of the respiration is increased after a meal ; and if he eats heartily or there be much dyspepsia, there is marked dyspnœa.

The shallowness of respiration is determined both by the general movement of the chest, and the amount of air inspired as shown by the spirometer.

On carefully looking in front of the exposed chest, it will commonly be seen that the breath motion is lessened over the whole thorax, but particularly at the upper part of it. This is well seen in women, in whom there is normally much motion at the upper part of the chest. It is not compensated by unusual abdominal respiration, as is found in conditions of disease in which there is an impediment to respiration, but the whole respiratory movement is lessened. When the spirometer is used (such an one as that arranged by us, which is capable of measuring even to one cubic inch of air, without offering any important impediment to respiration), it is found that the quantity of air which is inspired per minute is considerably lessened, so that if the person were in good health, he would inspire, in the sitting posture, at rest, 400 to 450 cubic inches per minute ; while he only actually inspires from 250 to 350 cubic inches in his ordinary mode of respiration. When this defect is multiplied by the twenty-four hours, it will be more clearly shown how great it is ; but the whole loss is not ascertained until the effect of exertion is imported into the question.

We have elsewhere given, in a tabular form,[1] the results which we have obtained in our experiments upon the effect of various kinds of exertion over the quantity of air inspired in health, and from these we learn that, taking the quantity inspired when lying and at rest as unity, the effect of ordinary exertion is as follows :—

TABLE No. 7.

Showing the influence of Exertion over the Quantity of Air inspired.

1. Lying .	1 0
2. Sitting	1.18
3. Standing	1.33
4. Singing, and reading aloud	1.26
5. Walking, at 1 mile per hour .	1.9
6. " 2 miles per hour .	2.76
7. " 3 "	3.22
8. " 4 "	5.0
9. Horse exercise—Walking	2.2
10. " Cantering	3.16
11. " Trotting	4.05
12. Running at 6 miles per hour .	7.0

Hence all men in health occupy a large portion of the day in exercises which increase the respiration from two to fourfold during the period of exertion, and when this is added to the respiration at rest, it greatly increases the total daily quantity. But in the cases now under consideration, not only is there inability or indisposition to take the exercise which is commonly taken in health, and thereby a large part of the ordinary increase is omitted, but during each moment of the day, whether at rest or with exertion, there is less respiration than occurs in health. Hence, when these two causes of decrease are considered together, we are enabled to form some conception of the importance of even a small but constant diminution in the respiration.

The feebleness of respiration is seen both in the ordinary and in forced respiration. In ordinary respiration, not only is the breath motion small, as it is also in chronic bronchitis, but the effort is feeble, and without that violence which is found in bronchitis. There appears to be not only less respiration, but less power to respire, as is evident to the most careless observer. In forced respiration it is, however, better marked, for it is much more difficult to train such an one than one in health to perform deep and slow respiration, both because the habit of shallow and feeble respiration

[1] Edinburgh Med. and Surg. Journ., Jan. 1850.

prevents him from duly apprehending what is required, and from his inability to inspire deeply. Such a person, when required to breathe deeply, performs quick and short acts of deeper inspiration, analogous to the short actions of a pair of hand-bellows when suddenly snatched open, or suddenly pressed down. The deep and slow inspiration which alone would fill the bellows (to continue the illustration), he does not easily apprehend and cannot readily perform. This we believe to be in part due to a forgetfulness of the proper habit of breathing, from the long continuance of an abnormal mode of breathing, and partly to inability to perform easily what is required. Moreover, it very often occurs, that when such an one is taking a deep inspiration, the inspiratory muscles too soon cease to act, and the chest suddenly falls to a certain extent, whilst he believes that he is still inspiring. This is most commonly seen in persons who are much enfeebled, and who, having led a very sedentary life, have not frequently evoked the full power of the inspiratory muscles. We have also found many cases in which the attempt at deep inspiration was frustrated by a sense of choking. This is readily accounted for, since in ordinary cases the sides of the pharynx, at the epiglottis, approach closely at the end of a deep inspiration, and when the sensibility is increased, such an effect is more likely to follow. We have seen the free edge of the epiglottis greatly contracted in such cases.

Feebleness and shallowness of the respiration are commonly associated, and we think that these two qualities must be taken together when considering their nature and effects, and that there is such a dependence of the one upon the other, that feeble breathing will induce shallow breathing.

The causes of this must be referred to those which ordinarily control breathing, viz., the muscular power and the nervous influence. Nothing need be advanced to prove that a feeble person does not breathe so powerfully and deeply as one in a vigorous state of health. This is seen universally, whatever may be the general disease in which the debility occurs, so that it would seem unnatural to find a feeble person breathing vigorously, and it is, in fact, due to the condition of the muscular system. We have already shown that in the conditions now under consideration there is a defective state of tonicity and power of the muscular system, and some amount of emaciation. But if we examine the chest of one not in the habit of using the lungs powerfully, it will be observed that both the pectoral muscles have lost some part of their bulk, and are become more or less thin and soft. Such is also the condition of the muscles of the back and the intercostals; and hence it is evident that, so far as the act of respiration depends upon the action of these muscles, it will be less efficiently performed; and inasmuch as we find a general condition of the muscular system which is exemplified in certain respiratory muscles which are external to the chest, so we may infer that the internal muscles have a similar defect of tone and power. Well-developed pectoral muscles and a vigorous state of the muscular system in general would be incompatible with feeble and shallow respiration ; and although in the state of disease now under consideration they do occasionally co-exist, they are exceptional conditions, and due to exceptional causes.

The association of shallowness and feebleness of respiration is seen in the most marked degree in tailors, shoemakers, clerks, and others who follow very sedentary occupations, and sit with the chest bent forwards. In such persons the act of respiration is at all times defective, and they are known to be very prone to the occurrence of phthisis. The stooping posture during employment is, however, far more common than the limits of this class would indicate; for in the inquiry upon 1000 phthisical persons engaged in a great variety of occupations, we found that 20 per cent. considered that it had been injurious to them.

Dyspnœa is not present in ordinary respiration.

It is well known that even in advanced cases of phthisis, dyspnœa is seldom complained of, except by those who are required to make muscular exertion, whilst at the same time the amount of air which is actually inspired and the power of respiration is considerably diminished. This is, no doubt, due to the facts that there may be great diminution in the vital capacity of the lungs without interfering with the small quantity of air which is inspired in ordinary respiration, to the lessened vital changes already referred to at page 41, and to the accommodation which the system has effected to the lessened capacity of respiration by the gradual diminution in the capacity of the lungs. Hence, *à fortiori*, we shall not expect to find dyspnœa in the early stages of phthisis, except when much respiratory effort is required, as in ascending steps, or running, or lifting weights. There are cases in which the respiration is aided by the patient locking his arms or hands behind his back, which gives increased power in the act of respiration by placing the relaxed pectoral muscles on the stretch, and enabling them to exercise their full powers as levers.

RATE OF RESPIRATION.

The rate of respiration is commonly somewhat increased, but, like that of pulsation, it is greatly influenced by the temperament of the patient. In the inquiry at the Hospital for Consumption before referred to, it varied in the different cases, on an average of 1500 observations, from 16 to 31 per minute, as recorded in Table No. 8 (page 69), in which the cases are arranged in the order of the rate of respiration. These refer to the disease in its various stages ; and whilst there is not so great diversity in cases in the early stage, there is yet considerable variation.

The importance of increased rapidity of respiration in conditions in which the respiration is shallow and feeble, is very evident, and analogous to that of rapidity with feebleness of circulation.

It is well established by the experiments of both Vierordt and ourself that, with lessened inspiration of air, there are lessened vital changes, and as the pulmonary circulation is in a great degree dependent upon the expansion and contraction of the lungs in the thoracic cavity, it is also certain that the diminution in the chest movements will physically render less free the pulmonary circulation directly, and the general circulation indirectly. Both of these actions proceed *pari passu*, and have equal importance. But when the respiratory movements are quickened, there is an increased quantity of air inhaled per minute, which will increase the vital changes, and, in a certain degree, sustain the circulation. Increased rapidity of respiration, when that function is performed in a feeble and shallow degree only, is the greatest advantage of which the condition is capable; and, like increase in the rate of pulsation, is beneficial, and only to be interfered with by increasing the completeness of the respiratory act. But there are cases in which the respiration is both incomplete in character and slow in repetition.

There is, as is well known, a correspondence between the rapidity of the respiration and that of the circulation; and whilst this is quite true when applied to cases in which the difference in rate is well marked, it does not admit of very close application. In our experiments in health we found, in an hourly inquiry through seventy-two consecutive hours in five persons,[1] the following number of pulsations to one respiration: Æt. 6, 4.5; æt. 8, 3.9; æt. 33, 4; æt. 36, 4.1; æt. 39, 3.4; and in another set[2] of investigations, carried on through eighteen hours of the day, the relation was—æt. 26, 4.63; æt. 33, 5; æt. 38, 5.25; and æt. 48, 5.72. In the inquiry in reference to phthisis (page 52), we arranged fourteen cases in the order of the rate of respiration and pulsation, and Table No. 9 (page 69), shows that the relative position under the two heads was, with one marked exception (85), somewhat similar. The numbers refer to the number of the cases in the hospital books.

VITAL CAPACITY.

This is, perhaps, a convenient occasion to refer to the vital capacity, or that amount of air which may be inspired from the extreme point of inspiration to the most complete expiration, or, if inspiration be tested, from the most complete expiration to the most complete inspiration. We would first remark, that this depends not only upon the condition of the lungs, but upon the power of respiration, the tact to perform the act perfectly, and the degree of action (spasmodic, perhaps) of the resisting muscles. We shall discuss the state of the lungs hereafter, and shall here only refer to the other condition.

The vital capacity of the lungs is diminished even when there are no evidences whatever of the presence of tubercular deposits.

We have tested this question with every care, and in many persons,

---

[1] Med.-Chir. Trans. 1856. [2] Phil. Trans. 1859.

and believe the proposition to be true in every period of the early stage of phthisis. No one will deny that the vital capacity is lessened where there is a material impediment to inspiration, such as occurs with deposited tubercle, but many may question it in the absence of this deposition, and affirm that, if it exist, there must also be the tubercle. We shall discuss this part of the subject in a future chapter, but here we affirm that there is a considerable diminution in the vital capacity, when there is no evidence whatever of the existence of any deposit.

The amount of diminution varies with the duration of the disease, and other conditions; but we have known females, æt. twenty, who could inspire only 100 to 120 cubic inches, and men of medium height whose capacity did not exceed 150 cubic inches. To render these statements of value, it is necessary to compare them with the healthy standard; but here we meet with a serious difficulty. Drs. Hutchinson and Balfour, and others, have ascertained the average vital capacity with different heights of body, and we are invited to compare our cases with their return. But their averages were derived from great numbers of persons, some of whom necessarily presented a vital capacity much above, and others as much below, this average quantity; and we compare an individual case, not with an individual high, medium, or low case in each class, but with the average derived from the high, medium, and low combined. If we had an equal number of cases of disease, with the number taken in health, and we simply desired to determine the average in both cases, the results might be comparable; but it is evidently a fallacious course to apply an average from various quantities to an individual quantity. This is doubtless the fallacy of all averages, when they are applied as a test to any individual case; but it proves that the system of averages is not suited to such a purpose. It is quite evident that if in a case of disease we find a small vital capacity, we should be at liberty to compare it with those cases in the great average which offered a small capacity; but if we should find an identity in the results, it would be of no avail, for by the proposition the one case is one of disease, and the other of health. Hence we advise the greatest caution in comparing the results of individual cases with those obtained from large averages; and by this source of error we explain so much of that which all persons who practise spirometry have found fallacious in the system.

Regarding the cases under discussion absolutely, we find a small vital capacity, and a smaller one than occurs in health, but what value must we attach to this fact? It is too much the habit to regard lessened vital capacity as a permanent condition, whilst we venture to assert that it is often a temporary one, and one existing wherever there is long-continued lessening of the vital powers. We must not infer from the fact that the patient inspires only a given quantity, that the lungs could not admit a larger amount of air, for we have shown that the capability to inspire as fully as the lungs would admit depends upon important causes, apart from the structure of the lungs, some of which are irremediable for the moment, but remediable subsequently, whilst others show an improvement even during the examination. The power to inhale belongs to the former, and whilst it may be increased, it must increase by slow degrees. The appreciation of the right method of inspiring or expiring air, or, as it may be termed, the knack of respiring, may be acquired more and more perfectly during each examination; and so much is this the case, that no one would take the first attempt as indicating the true vital capacity. It is constantly found that the result will vary 10 to 40 cubic inches at different efforts, and as we teach the patient, and he clearly apprehends what is required, we find evidence of larger vital capacity. The same observation will also apply to the action of the muscles which impede extreme movements of the chest, whether in expiration or inspiration. No one can have been largely engaged in examination of his own respiration without being conscious of a sense of constriction at various parts of the chest, and especially about the diaphragm, when attention is given to the respiration, and it is quite impossible to overcome that resistance by any efforts of the will. It is only removed when the attention is withdrawn, or, in other words, when the person has acquired the free and natural method of breathing. If this be so with persons in health, who understand what is required, and who have had large personal experience, how much more will it apply to persons in disease, who are nervous and untrained in this kind of inquiry?

Hence we feel that there are many sources of variation in the results of spirometry, that until the case presents features which, in the hands of competent men, render spirometry unnecessary, we can seldom go beyond the fact of having ascertained the amount inspired, and must infer the cause of the supposed diminution with caution.

SPIROMETERS.

This would be a favourable opportunity on which to refer to the various instruments which are in use for the purpose of measuring the amount of air inspired, but as we do not attach great value to this investigation in cases of disease, when the case is under the observation of those well-trained in the physical examination of the chest, we shall not occupy much space in doing so.

The air-holder of Hutchinson is now familiarly known to the profession, and that of Pereira (which was devised after the apparatus arranged by Sir H. Davy) is of a similar nature, and both have the same merits and defects. They are arranged to measure expiration, and are graduated to 400 or 500 cubic inches, which is more than enough for the largest expiration. They are so counterpoised as rather to favour the ascent of the inverted holder as it rises from the water, but there is no sufficient attempt to exactly balance the weight of the holder at different elevations. Hence, whilst they are sufficiently accurate for the purpose now under consideration, they cannot be regarded as instruments fitted for exact scientific research.

A modification of this spirometer has been made by M. Schnepf, so that by varying the weight of the chain in its different parts, it becomes a travelling counterpoise; and the weight of the holder is so exactly balanced in every part of its course, that stopcocks and corrections become unnecessary. We insert a drawing of this, the least imperfect of this kind of spirometer.

Dr. Lewis, of Caermarthen, has recently introduced a very simple and cheap instrument, which fulfils the required indications with a sufficient degree of accuracy. The principle of its construction is the displacement of a volume of water equal to that of the air expired. The apparatus consists of a large glass jar, placed on its side at an angle, so as to favour the removal of the fluid, and furnished with an index, large tubes, and mouthpiece. When the graduation of such an instrument is carefully made, it becomes so far a perfect instrument, and the only defect to which we need to refer is the resistance which the mass of water offers to the expiratory force; and although this is very appreciable at the end of expiration, when the force is greatly reduced, we are of opinion, after careful trial, that its indications

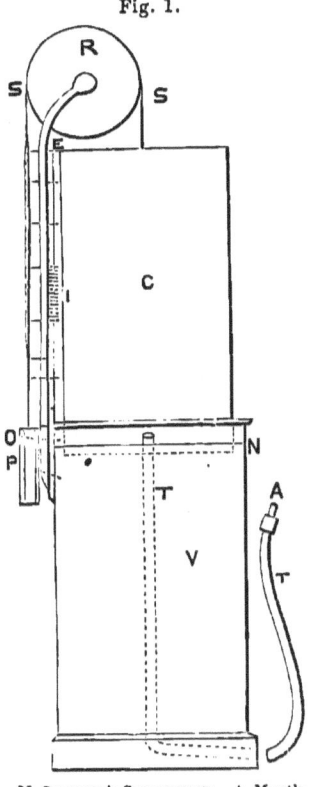

Fig. 1.

M. Schnepf's Spirometer.—A. Mouthpiece. C. Inverted Receiver. E. Scale. P. Counterpoise. R. Wheel. S. Chain. T. Tube, open above the water-line inside, and ending at A outside. V. Cistern to contain water.

are as reliable as those of much more expensive instruments. The following drawing has been kindly furnished by Dr. Lewis:—

The spirometer which we have used in our various inquiries, is an inverted dry gas meter of improved construction, which has been adapted to measure the air in inspiration, and to register from one to one million cubic inches. It will, therefore, indicate the quantity of air inhaled at one full inspiration, as required in the determination of the vital capacity, or it will register the number of cubic inches inspired during ordinary respiration in an hour, or indeed for any period, however long or short.   It is manufactured by Messrs. Croll, Rait, and Co., Kingsland Road, N. E.

Fig. 2.

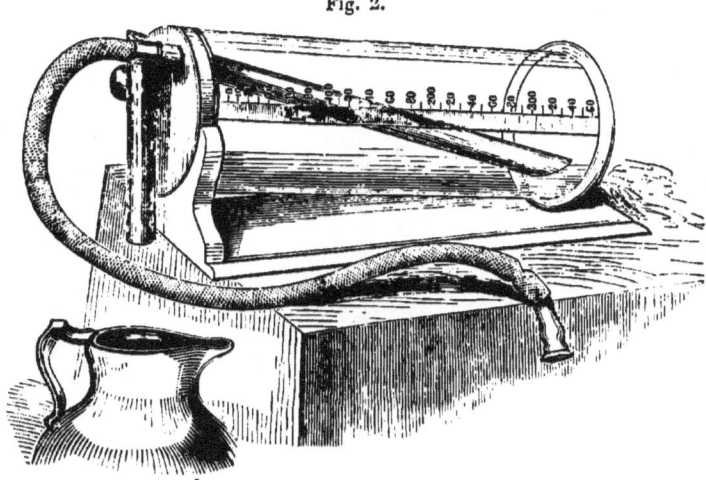

For the further discussion of this subject, we must refer to a series of papers on the spirometer published by us in the *Medical Circular* of 1857.

CHAPTER XII.

INNERVATION.

Innervation is commonly lessened.

We are not able to enter at any length into the question of inner-vation, since the subject is at present too much involved in mystery to enable us to do more than indicate the general principles involved in that act.

There can be no doubt that, whilst there may be certain powers in-herent in tissues, as, for example, in the muscular and fibrous tissues, there is a separate controlling influence, which not only calls forth the full power of action of each tissue and organ, but co-ordinates movements, and enables the body to act in its various parts simulta-neously and as a harmonious whole. This, whatever it may be, acts through the nervous system, and hence a primary and controlling power is given to that system.

The amount of power which may thus be exerted varies with different conditions of the system, so that at one time the nervous force appears to be efficient, and the responses of the tissues which it calls into action are ready and effectual, whilst in others one or both of these conditions of force are weakened, and the resulting action is below the standard of health, without there having been any serious injury inflicted upon the nervous centres. This is seen particularly in conditions of mal-nutrition from any cause, and as nutrition is doubtless greatly under the control of the nervous influence, we are brought to argue in a circle, and to show that nervous influence sustains the nutritive act, and is itself in part dependent upon the degree of efficiency of nutrition.

So far as the defective nutrition, with its host of consequences, may be a sure guide, it is safe to affirm that there is lessened inner-vation in the early stage of phthisis, and as that condition carries in its train nearly every feature of the disease, we think we are warranted in affirming that it is the ordinary condition of the nerv-ous system. With lessened appetite for food, lessened accumulation of food, more ready elimination of fluid, mal-nutrition, lessened muscular tone and force, lessened cardiac force, and feeble respira-tion, there must also be lessened innervation, whether we regard the latter as a consequence or a cause of some of the former.

We have now discussed some of the larger and more general ques-tions which affect the health of the body and are concerned in the production of phthisis, such as mental activity, assimilation, calorifica-tion, elimination, circulation, respiration, and innervation; and now proceed to discuss others of a subordinate and less general character, and which cannot be arranged under any common heading.

CHAPTER XIII.

THE MENSES AND LEUCORRHŒA.

The menstrual function is frequently disturbed, but probably not in a greater degree than occurs in health. There is much liability to leucorrhœa.

When we consider the large mass of cases in the disease now under discussion, we think that this proposition is true: but for a due estimation of the importance of the irregularity, it is essential to ascertain the frequency of its occurrence in health. We can scarcely enter upon the consideration of the menstrual function beyond the statement of the facts, for the physiology is at present too obscure to enable us to afford the explanations which we desire. It is well known that, in the advanced stages of the disease, it is usual to find that the menses have ceased; and, on the other hand, in young women, in whom the functions of the body are not vigor-

ously performed, whether temporarily or for a long period, it is very
common to find a deficiency or an arrest of the menstrual flow ; but
in neither case can we afford a sufficient explanation of the fact. To
say that they are associated with general debility and enervation,
or are dependent in part upon the degree of activity of the body in
the occupation of life, is simply to state co-ordinate facts, and does
not in the least explain them, and yet such is nearly all that we can
adduce in reference to this matter.

We have thought it would be of interest and importance to inquire into the natural tendencies of the system in reference to this
function in phthisical persons, with a view to ascertain if any special
predisposition existed in them, and particularly to inquire as to the
age at which the menses first appeared, and the general degree of
regularity of the menstrual function during health, and we therefore
instituted an inquiry upon 1000 out-patients for that purpose. The
result showed that the epoch of menstruation occurred at from seven
to twenty-four years of age, and the proportionate appearance of
the menses at each age was ascertained to be as follows :—

TABLE No. 10.

Showing the Age at the First Appearance of the Menses.

Æt. years.				Per Cent.	Æt. years.				Per Cent.
7	.	.	.	.26	16	.	.	.	15.1
10	.	.	.	.53	17	.	.	.	8.0
11	.	.	.	4.4	18	.	.	.	6.0
12	.	.	.	6.2	19	.	.	.	3.9
13	.	.	.	11.4	20	.	.	.	1.3
14	.	.	.	18 2	21	.	.	.	.26
15	.	.	.	18.2	24	.	.	.	.26

It therefore appears that æt. 14 and 15 was the most frequent
period of the appearance of the menses, and that there was a progressive increase from æt. eleven, and a decrease until æt. twenty
years. It is improbable that so large a number as $11\frac{1}{2}$ per cent. of
the women in this climate have the menses previous to or at æt.
twelve, and hence, perhaps, there may be a slight preponderance
in favour of the phthisical patients; but since more than 60 per cent.
of the latter commenced to menstruate at thirteen, fourteen, fifteen,
and sixteen years of age, it is highly probable that no important
peculiarity existed in them. We also ascertained that in 4 per
cent. the menses had never appeared, although they had all passed
the usual period of the commencement of that function.

The same patients have also furnished us with information as to
the degree of regularity with which this function had been performed
in the course of the life *previous* to the commencement of phthisis,
and we found that there was a tendency to deficiency in the menses.
The menstrual discharge was excessive in 6 per cent., and too
frequent in 2.52 per cent., but it was deficient in quantity in 29
per cent., and with the intervals too prolonged in 6.7 per cent. In

reference to the combinations of these conditions in the same person, it may be of interest to remark, that in 15.2 per cent. the discharge was insufficient and too seldom, in 1.2 per cent. it was excessive and too frequent, in .5 per cent. it was excessive and too seldom, and in .25 per cent. it was insufficient and too frequent.

Hence we are entitled to state that the menstrual function has been well established in the great majority of cases of phthisis, and is performed with tolerable regularity during the period of health. It evinces a distinct tendency to deficiency in quantity, and in only a few cases is there an excessive discharge. We have also met with many instances in which there is much suffering at, or immediately preceding the monthly recurrences of the menses, and in such the discharge was commonly deficient, and the duration restricted to one or two days. In others, gastralgia of a severe kind has occurred at the same periods, and in many instances hæmoptysis has preceded the monthly period, or has appeared during the week when the menses have been deficient.

Whilst, therefore, we find that there are numerous evidences of a disturbed state of the menstrual function existing during health in cases of early phthisis, we cannot at present affirm that they occur more frequently than in other enfeebled organizations. We are, however, convinced that there is no further disturbance induced by the disease in question in its early stage, but whenever, and to whatever, degree it occurs, it demands a remedy.

The predisposition to the occurrence of leucorrhœa is certainly marked. In the period preceding the development of phthisis, not less than 45.6 per cent. of the cases already referred to, had been liable to the discharge, and this disposition is still further increased by duration of time and the occurrence of the phthisical symptoms. It is also very common to find this state associated with deficiency in the menstrual function, and particularly in unmarried women of sedentary habits and lymphatic temperament.

CHAPTER XIV.

MUSCULAR PAINS.

Muscular pains about the chest are very common.

There is another local condition to which we must direct attention, which often precedes any evidence of the early stage of phthisis, and very frequently attends its course, viz., myalgia both in the front and back of the chest. The most frequent seats of this affection are the pectoral muscles and the muscles attached to the base and inferior angle of the scapula. The former are very variable in degree and seat, and seldom remain fixed in any place. They are commonly uninfluenced by exertion, but sometimes the movement of the arm causes pain. The latter are more commonly found between the shoulders and at the inferior angle of the scapula than at any other part; and whilst the former are far more common in men, the latter are far more frequent in women.

The nature of these pains has been more correctly understood of late years than formerly, and we owe it in no small degree to the vigorous mind and acute observation of Dr. Inman, whose treatise upon this subject is worthy of careful study. These are not attended by any febrile disturbance of the general system, and are not usually acute, but sometimes the pain is very urgent, and is much increased on deep inspiration. In the latter cases we should formerly have diagnosed pleuritis; but whilst such might be correct in some instances, it is more probable that it is a muscular pain, induced by calling the muscles into action. In the disease now under discussion we need not entertain much fear as to the diagnosis; for whether it be in any severe case localized pleuritis or severe myalgia, the effect of treatment will be equally satisfactory.

The relations of this myalgia are often obscure, but so far as we have been able to apprehend them, they are very important. The connection with exertion, and the atonicity of the muscle, which is commonly found in the early stage of phthisis, may be excluded from these observations, for they are commonly plain; but there are other causes of very frequent occurrence. In reference to men, we have often found them in persons addicted to onanism, or who have been so in former years. In such persons myalgia of the chest is a most frequent occurrence, and although not severe, it attracts the attention of the patient, and leads him to fear more important mischief. We shall recur to this subject at a future page.

In other cases, in which this cause cannot be discovered, we have found chest myalgia of the moderate degree, and intermitting, before any other condition of the early stage of phthisis has occurred; and as such often remain long under treatment, we have had the opportunity of tracing the addition of symptom to symptom, until the evidences of the early stage of phthisis are before us. Whether this is simply one of the numerous conditions which are due to pre-existent influences, or whether it may be regarded in any way as inducing other evidences of early phthisis, we cannot determine; but there can be no doubt that persistent or often-recurring myalgia of the inspiratory and expiratory muscles will tend to a diminution in the action of these organs, either by rendering inspiration inefficient or by unduly limiting expiration, and thereby lessen the chest movements; a condition which, as we shall show, is essentially connected with the early stage of phthisis. We incline to the latter view, and in doing so shall err on the safe side; for it will at least show us how important it is to adopt every method which may cause their speedy removal.

CHAPTER XV.

THE THROAT.

The form of the throat in phthisis is peculiar, and differs much from that seen in chronic bronchitis.

We discussed the conditions of the throat in phthisis and bronchitis in a paper published in the *Liverpool Medical Journal* for 1857—a journal which is now defunct. In that communication we pointed out that there is ordinarily a condition of the throat in phthisis quite different from that which is found in chronic bronchitis.

On inspecting the throat in an ordinary case of phthisis, it will be seen that the fauces are generally narrow and small, and the anterior arch has nearly disappeared, whilst the posterior remains largely developed. The cavity between the arches is large and deep, and the tonsillar mucous follicles are frequently enlarged. The whole structures are attenuated, and present a sharp outline. The pillars of the posterior arches are commonly large, and project into the cavity of the pharynx during forcible expiratory efforts. The movements of the throat in inspiration and expiration are normal, but those which attend the contraction of the pharynx at its lower part seem to be increased in vigour, for the lateral contraction which they induce about the epiglottis is very considerable. But in ordinary cases of old bronchitis the cavity of the fauces is very wide; there is no attenuation of the parts, and the respiratory movements of the throat are greatly diminished, as may be seen during forced expiration, in the manner exhibited in the drawing on page 87.

There is commonly a state of hyperæsthesia of the throat.

We believe that but few cases occur in which there is not some complaint made of the throat, such as is represented by the word tickling, or irritation. This, in many instances, is very slight, so that it is ascertained only after inquiry; and in nearly all cases it is a condition which varies in intensity, and is oftentimes entirely absent for a certain period.

The conditions of the throat which are commonly found are two:—

First.—A state of pallor of the whole mucous membrane, with an attenuated state of the arches and the pillars of the pharynx, and an evident sulcus in the intervals between the pillars. It also frequently occurs that the pharynx is contracted at its upper part, either antero-posteriorly, or laterally, or in the whole circle, so that the poste-

rior wall of the pharynx seems to be brought very near to the root
of the tongue (when the latter is well depressed and inspiration is
effected by the mouth), and the uvula seems to fall nearly upon the
posterior wall, or the whole aperture is greatly contracted, and
with difficulty can the patient be persuaded to inhale a full volume
of air by the mouth. In all cases of this class the uvula is not elongated, but on the contrary, if at all changed, it is rather retracted;
and when the sense of irritation is very considerable, there will be
found more or less froth or foam over the whole throat. In this
condition there is a sense of constriction in breathing, and sometimes
in swallowing, and great sensitiveness to excitants as the spatula,
finger, or cold air. When the whole aperture is contracted, the
cough is oftentimes of a spasmodic character, and noisy.

Second.—The condition now known as follicular disease, in which
the simple epithelial glands, which are abundant on the posterior
wall of the pharynx, become enlarged and vascular, and present the
appearance of small flattened red currants. In this condition there
is not unusually, but yet not necessarily, some elongation of the uvula,
and a little suffusion of the mucous membrane of the whole fauces,
with enlarged vessels upon the back and sides, and sometimes also
some enlargement of the tonsils. There are not, however, in these
signs any evidences of inflammatory action, neither is the sense of
irritation, or of choking, so acute and urgent as in many cases of
the anæmic throat, but there is a moderate degree of irritation, and
it is persistent. It also frequently happens that the tongue is loaded
in this condition of the throat, both in health and disease, whilst in
the anæmic throat the tongue is usually clean, or covered only with
froth, or a very thin white covering.

In a few cases, we find a little thickening of the whole mucous
lining of the throat, without any exaltation of colour, and with diminution rather than increase of sensibility; but these are conditions
which belong to the scrofulous diathesis rather than to the disease
which we have now under consideration. In the condition of the
throat common to the early stage of phthisis it may be affirmed that
exaltation of sensibility is usually met with.

On examining the throat in either of the above-mentioned conditions, it is essential that the patient be placed before a good light,
that the throat be below the level of the observer, that the tongue
be well laid down by the broad spatula pressed firmly, but without
any approach to violence; and, above all, that the patient inspire
by the mouth and not by the nose. Some of these conditions are
difficult of attainment; for it very often happens that the patient
cannot be induced so to expand the lips as to allow the light to freely
enter the throat, or the presence of the spatula near the root of the
tongue excites irritation; or, lastly, that the patient will persist in
holding the breath during the examination instead of breathing at
the normal rate, and thus limits the duration of the examination, and
induces a sense of sickness. The opening of the lips may be effected,

and the presence of the spatula be tolerated by a little care and perseverance; but until the patient can be induced to open the throat, and breathe quietly with the spatula in the mouth, it will be impossible to make a satisfactory examination. For the latter purpose, it is advisable to close the patient's nose, so that being compelled to breathe through the mouth, the back part of the tongue may fall from the *velum palati*, and the patient be conscious of the air passing down the throat by the mouth, and when this has been attained, it will generally occur that the patient can be induced to continue the respiration by the mouth; or it may sometimes suffice to induce the patient before the spatula is used, to inhale deeply by the mouth, so as to feel the presence of the current of cool air in the pharynx when entering by the mouth in a large volume, and so learn what it is to inhale by the mouth and not by the nose. It is needless to say that so long as inspiration is effected by the nose, the tongue is raised and closes the mouth, and no investigation of the pharynx can be made.

It is also to be commended so to depress the tongue as to expose the upper edge of the epiglottis—not that there is commonly a condition about that part of the pharynx which is not seen somewhat higher—but to expose the epiglottis implies that the pharynx has been well explored. It is not to be understood that there is any real difficulty in seeing the upper edge of the epiglottis in ordinary cases; but, on the contrary, if the head be held moderately backward, and the back part of the tongue pressed firmly downwards and forwards, the epiglottis is at once exposed. There are, however, some cases in which the sensibility of the parts, or the wilfulness of the patient, prevents the use of the necessary pressure, at least for a time; and there are others in which the epiglottis is so low in the throat, that, with every facility and effort, it cannot be well seen. The last case is, however, rare, the second is not by any means common, so that the former cases are those which will ordinarily engage attention.

The importance of a condition of hyperæsthesia of the pharynx has no reference to the structure of the throat itself, or to the due performance of its functions, but in its relation to the occurrence of cough, and the action of cold air in inspiration.

CHAPTER XVI.

COUGH.

There is commonly only a small or moderate amount of coughing.
Coughing is essentially a reflex act, and is due to eccentric irritation, but the irritation may be applied directly to the true seat of the act, or be transmitted from distant organs. In the act of cough-

ing, the following conditions must exist. 1st. Closure of the larynx at its upper orifice. 2d. Suspension of the respiratory movements. 3d. Tension of the thorax by contraction of the muscles, and particularly of the diaphragm and the abdominal muscles, during which act the air is displaced, and the upper lobes are distended by pressure from below. And, 4th. Sudden opening of the larynx, and forcible ejection of the previously confined and compressed air. As a subordinate action, the circulation, both pulmonic and systemic, is interfered with, and during a fit of coughing the pulsation is much accelerated.

The importance of the pharynx in the act of coughing may be seen in the immediate production of that act on the application of any irritating body to the posterior and lateral walls, and also by the rapid and violent contraction of the cavity which occurs in the first part of the act of coughing. When the pressure upon the lungs from below is exerted by the abdominal muscles and the diaphragm, the larynx is simultaneously raised about half an inch; the root of the tongue is carried upwards and backwards, and the posterior wall of the pharynx is brought forwards, so that the posterior aspect of the epiglottis is in approximation to the anterior aspect of the posterior wall of the pharynx; and this, together with the circular contraction of the pharynx about the epiglottis, closes the apertures both of the pharynx and larynx. This was shown by us in 1857, and the engraving opposite was published afterwards in the *Journal de Physiologie.*

It has also been affirmed that during this action the chordæ vocales are brought into apposition and the chink of the glottis is closed; but that the true closure of the larynx during the act of coughing does not take place there, or at least is not entirely there, may be proved by the circumstances attending ulceration of the free edge of the epiglottis, when, as is well known, the patient cannot cough at all, and the sharp sound accompanying the emission of the air is lost, and a dull sound of air rushing through an imperfectly closed aperture attends the attempt to cough. This inability is due to the absence of the elastic substance which, when present and applied to the wall of the pharynx, closes the aperture of the larynx. It is also of great interest to remark that, immediately before free inspiration is effected, during the choking which follows the application of the strong solution of caustic to the pharynx, there is commonly a sudden eructation of air from the œsophagus, proving that with the apnœa there was closure of the pharynx at its lower extremity, as above described. Hence, there is reason to believe that the pharynx is the essential seat of cough.

But it is believed that irritation set up in other and distant parts produces cough also, as, for example, in the bronchi, the pulmonary structure, or even in the stomach. It is, however, to be borne in mind that the degree of irritation as a cause of cough which is observed when foreign bodies have passed through the larynx into the bronchi is by no means so great as is observed when irritants are directly applied to the pharynx; also, that the amount of cough bears no relation to the amount of irritation existing below the larynx, and that stomach affections usually exist without producing any cough. When cough is owing to these causes it occurs through reflex action upon the pharynx, and hence in all cases it is proper to regard the pharynx as the true seat of this expiratory act. The importance of this question is evident, both with regard to the causes and the treatment of cough, and to these we shall have further occasion to refer.

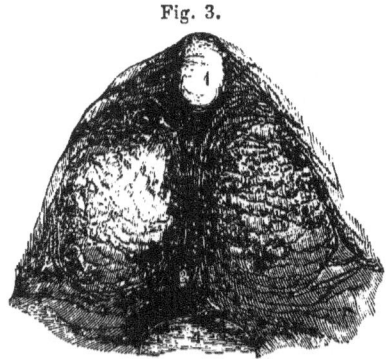

Fig. 3.

DRAWING OF THE PHARYNX IN ITS CONTRACTED STATE, AS DURING THE FIRST PART OF THE ACT OF COUGHING.—1. Uvula contracted, and drawn upwards. 2. Tonsils drawn forwards and inwards. 3. Pharynx drawn forwards and inwards, and corrugated into folds. 4. Upper edge of epiglottis rendered convex, and applied to the posterior wall of the pharynx.

As we have already shown that there is hyperæsthesia of the pharynx in a large number of cases of early phthisis, it follows that there will be a tendency to the occurrence of cough, and the amount of cough will (within certain limits), be in proportion to the amount of hyperæsthesia. As a general observation it may, however, be stated, that at the period in question the amount of cough is not usually a distressing feature in the case.

The nature of the cough is commonly short, and repeated a few times at each attack. It is not usually violent or causing much succussion, but sometimes it is spasmodic. It more frequently occurs on moving into a cooler atmosphere, as on going into the hall from the warm sitting room, or out of doors, or into the bedroom at night, and is consequently more frequent on taking out of door exercise, and at night. It is also immediately excited when, with a hot and perspiring skin, the clothes are suddenly removed, or cold air gains access by any means. It is not unfrequently irritable in the early morning, and especially soon after rising, and doubtless from a similar cause, for at that period of the day the temperature is commonly low. It is also worse in the colder seasons of the year, as the end of autumn, the winter, and the early spring, and is then more frequent throughout the day. A dry frost, however, although it causes cough, is not so constant a cause as a cold and raw atmosphere, and particularly one in which there is fog and smoke, and the latter condition is perhaps the most injurious of any in which such a patient could be placed. All these influences seem to have one common mode of attack, namely, the inhalation of air which irritates by the temperature or other qualities, and the effect is always greater in proportion to the volume of air inspired, the intensity of

those qualities, and the sensibility of the mucous surface over which
the air passes.

There are also numerous cases in which the cough is increased
after meals. Such are commonly instances in which there is much
general sensibility of the nervous system, and of the pharynx in
particular, and in which the vital capacity of the lungs is much
diminished; but in many instances it is due to food which produces
irritation as it passes over the pharynx, or remains in small particles
attached to it, or excites the reflex action from the stomach to which
we have referred. The cause of this cough is not at all times easy
of detection, but we have been accustomed to seek it in two directions:
1st. It will manifestly arise if the food mechanically irritate the
sensitive mucous membrane of the pharynx, whether by being in
large lumps from imperfect mastication, or containing condiments,
as pepper, salt, or mustard, or possessing inherent stimulating qualities, as spirits, or remain adherent to the membrane from an imperfect deglutition, or from the absence of fluid following the deglutition
of solid food; and all these conditions are remediable. 2d. It has
appeared to us to have some connection with a diminution of the
capacity of the thorax which follows a full meal, by the distended
stomach pressing the diaphragm upwards, and impeding respiration;
or it may be in part due to the fulness of the bloodvessels, and the
increased innervation which follows a meal, in which the pharynx
partakes in common with other parts of the internal organs. The
point to which we desire especially to call attention, is, that the
cough is not usually or necessarily associated with the condition of
the lungs, to which we shall have hereafter to particularly refer;
but whatever may be the immediate source of irritation, the seat of
the cough is for the most part located within our reach.

CHAPTER XVII.

EXPECTORATION.

There is commonly a small amount of expectoration.

In referring to the nature and quantity of the expectoration, it is
necessary to premise that we discuss only those which commonly
occur in the course of the disease, and not such temporary conditions
as may be found in persons in health, or in every condition of
disease.

The quantity of secretion expectorated is very small, and does
not exceed from one-quarter to one-half ounce in the twenty-four
hours. It usually occurs in the early morning and after meals, and
follows a certain amount of cough which then prevails. During the

other periods of the day its appearance is quite uncertain, and does not attract attention; but it is always associated with cough.

The nature of the expectoration is very uniform, except in the temporary condition of cold, &c., which we have excluded from consideration. It is semi-transparent, or only very slightly opaque, and not unfrequently shows lines or small masses of darker colour. It is never uniformly yellowish, greenish, or pinkish, and when these colours are found they are due to other conditions. There is no form to the sputa, but it is glairy and irregular in shape, according to the place in which it is deposited, and sometimes is very tenacious. A frothy condition is not necessary, but when it is found, it is due to irritation of the pharynx, with much cough, or is associated with bronchitis.

On microscopic examination, it is found to consist of a glairy, semi-translucent matrix, in which are found tessellated epithelial cells, whole or in parts, and frequently with large cells, of a black colour, filled with nuclei and granules. There is not, we believe, any of the yellow elastic structure of the lungs found at this stage, for we are now concerned with an earlier condition than that of destruction of the lung tissue; and although the expectoration of lung tissue may be associated with the signs and symptoms which belong to the early stage of phthisis, there will usually be other evidences which prove that the disease has progressed further than the point under inquiry. It is believed that cases occur in which destruction of the lung tissue is found in a very small part of the lung only, whilst all the other parts retain their normal structure and function; but to this we venture to demur. We believe that all such cases exhibit, and have long exhibited, in the lungs, the signs of an earlier stage, and that with such general signs there will be superadded, in progress of time, deposition, and then destruction, and both may be localized in a small space; but such are truly cases of more advanced disease.

The cases in which there must be doubt as to the existence of localized destruction of lung are very few, comparatively, except those which are complicated with other diseases, which cause respiratory sounds fitted to prevent a careful examination of the chest for the detection of the softening in question, as, for example, in cases of continued bronchitis; but, without entering further into the argument, we exclude the cases in which yellow elastic tissue is found in the sputa, without acute inflammatory action, from those now under discussion.

The *chief* sources of the secretion in the early stage of phthisis are the fauces and pharynx. The tonsils emit a secretion of a glairy nature, and having the characters above described. When there is much sensibility of the pharynx, and cough, the surface of the mucous membrane is covered with minute bubbles of air, inclosed in a very small quantity of mucus, which are ejected from time to time; and when there is enlargement of the mucous follicles, each

5

hypertrophied body secretes a glairy fluid with detached epithelial scales, which is abundant according to the number and activity of the follicles. But, besides these, it frequently occurs that secretions, passing over from the nares, rest upon the pharynx, cause cough, and are expectorated by the mouth. It is scarcely possible to examine the upper part of the pharynx frequently without being struck with the amount of secretion which is often found lying upon the membrane. This has a character different from that which we have described, since it is opaque, and contains many mucous cells and some granular matter. Ciliated epithelium will also be often found in this secretion, for that form of epithelium lines nearly the whole nares, and covers the nasal aspect of the soft palate and the nasal end of the pharynx; but it gives place to the tessellated epithelium above mentioned in the lower part of the pharynx. The secretion from the nares is, we believe, often mistaken for that which is presumed to occur from the bronchi, trachea, and larynx, in which places the ciliated epithelium again appears. It must be borne in mind that in many persons the nasal secretion is very abundant, and a large portion of it passes into the pharynx; and all persons are conscious that a certain amount is thus disposed of in perfect health.

It may be again remarked, that the seat of cough is particularly that part in which there is tessellated epithelium, and in which there are but insufficient means whereby either particles of food, or such accumulation of secretion, may be detached from it. Hence cough is the natural remedy for the defect.

CRETACEOUS EXPECTORATION.

There are cases numerous, yet few comparatively, in which we find the expectoration of white chalky-looking particles which, when taken between the fingers in the fresh state, rub down, and make an opaque granular fluid, such as would occur when a small portion of softened chalk was rubbed with mucus. When they have been separated from the sputa and allowed to dry, they appear to be small roughish granules of a white color, opaque, and resembling chalk somewhat disintegrated. They vary in size, but usually are twice or thrice the size of a pin's head, and sometimes they are equal in size to half a split pea, or even larger.

Since the comparatively recent researches into the nature of tubercle and of tubercular phthisis, it was common to notice substances in the sputa of consumptives which resembled particles of boiled rice, and to describe them as portions of eliminated tuberculous matter in some of its secondary processes. As knowledge has increased, we have looked with increasing distrust upon the relationship of these matters to tubercle, and, indeed, their importance has almost passed away, either from the small attention which is now paid to the expectoration in relation to the daily examinations which were made thirty years ago; from the small importance which is attached to such matters, either in elucidating or in treating the disease ; or from the grave doubts which are entertained as to their connection with tubercle. We think that, perhaps in the present day we err in giving so little attention to the sputa, and thus allow matters to pass unnoticed which should excite interest, but we fully partake in the general doubts which are now extended to these substances.

The cretaceous matters which are expectorated seem to rest upon more tangible grounds, inasmuch as we do not see any other source for them than that to which they are referred. Yet it must be borne in mind, that as yet we have no proof as to their nature. When they are placed under the microscope they exhibit simply a mineral character, without any vital structure whatever, except epithelial scales. It is true that, admitting their nature to be as assumed, such would be the case, because they have passed through the stage in which they were vital structures, and are become secondary degenerations with mineral matter. There are some *primâ facie* objections to this reasoning, since in no case do we find precisely similar bodies in the lungs, whilst they are not unfrequently found in the glands; and although there may be a probability as to their origin, it rests not upon established facts.

It is also worthy of note that these matters are rarely expectorated in cases in which the disease proceeds to a fatal termination, but in such as offer none or but very questionable evidence of the disease, or in which the presumed disease is manifestly connected with bronchitis. They are regarded as the evidence of a healthy process in parts of the lungs which are presumed to have been afflicted with tubercular deposition. Now, in the absence of proof as to the pre-existent condition of the lungs—proof which can rarely be obtained—and bearing in mind the few instances in which they occur, and also the rarity of true tubercular disease being arrested after destruction of the tissue has begun, it will become us rather to look out for some other source of this matter than an ordinary tubercular deposit in the tissues which commonly proceeds to a fatal termination. We are not able to give further information as to them, but we entertain doubts as to their nature and supposed site in the lungs. Assuming them to be of the nature assigned to them, we think that they must be admitted to occur in the class of cases under discussion, for there can be no doubt that many cases with this kind of expectoration, are in apparent health, or regain their health; and it is no answer to this statement, that in others tubercular disease does manifest itself and pursue its fatal course, because the very great frequency of tubercular disease renders it probable that it will occur occasionally, or even frequently in every condition. We have met with them in every stage and condition of the disease—in the advanced cases, with profuse expectoration, in which there is no hope of arresting the disease, in cases in which the phthisical symptoms were marked by co-existent and long-continued bronchitis, and in instances in which the most minute and careful examination of the lungs led to the belief that no disease existed, but it would be of no value to cite the cases in detail.

CHAPTER XVIII.

HÆMOPTYSIS.

In a majority of cases there has been hæmoptysis in some degree, but not necessarily proceeding from the lungs.

There is much want of uniformity in the cases of early phthisis as to the occurrence of hæmoptysis, the frequency of the occurrence, and its supposed cause; but there is more uniformity as to the quantity of blood which is expectorated. It is well known that there are many cases in which the disease proceeds to a fatal termination without hæmoptysis having occurred, and others in which there is very considerable destruction of the lung tissue, and no discharge of blood appears until a yet later period. In the inquiry upon 1,000 patients in the second and third stages of phthisis, we found that one-third, viz., 32.2 per cent. of the females, and 33 per cent. of the males, had never had the slightest hæmoptysis. Such cases are, however, the exceptions to the general rule, that hæmoptysis is common at some period in the progress of phthisis.

There may be a difference in opinion upon this point, according as we include the appearance of very small streaks of blood, even at distant periods, or only such quantities as have attracted the attention of the patient, and which, from the proximity of the occurrences to the supposed period of the commencement of the disease, may be more closely associated with it. We are accustomed, in our inquiries into this matter, to notice the occurrence of hæmoptysis in two degrees, viz., slight or streaks, and large quantities, but to note only, or chiefly, the period of its first occurrence; and whilst believing that the impression to be produced upon the mind in reference to the prognosis should vary with any great difference in the quantity of blood lost, we believe that the most important period to be noticed is that of the first occurrence, from whatever cause; and that it will not avail us, or it will beg the question, to attempt to exclude all occurrences which, in our opinion, had no connection with the disease.

Commonly, the quantity of blood expectorated is very small, and amounts only to a streak in one or only a few quantities of the sputa. It is usually noticed on one occasion only at a time, and may have appeared on one, two or three occasions. Sometimes the first occasion of it is somewhat sudden, and there is a so-called mouthful of blood spat at once, and probably no return follows; but in a few cases there is profuse hemorrhage on one or perhaps two occasions, amounting to some ounces, or, as is stated, to a pint, and occurring with coughing, but without any noticeable effort. The latter accident is so impressed upon the memory in such cases, that the patient commonly dates the commencement of his disease from that period; and it not unfrequently happens that it occurred some years before, and the health was believed to have been subsequently quite restored. These, although the most noticeable of all the cases, are yet few, and quite exceptional; and it may be affirmed as a general rule, that whilst hæmoptysis occurs in a majority of the cases of early phthisis, the quantity is very small, and does not exceed a few streaks or specks.

This fact has long been admitted, and because it is general and well established, great importance has been attached to it in the diagnosis of the disease. Let us, therefore, inquire what is the precise value of such an occurrence, what is its seat, and to what is it usually owing?

Those who attach importance to the occurrence of this small amount of hæmoptysis, do not now do so on account of the loss of blood, although Cullen in his *Synopsis*, page 83, introduces the alarming sentence: " The consequence of hæmoptysis is PHTHISIS, emaciation, debility, cough, hectic fever, and in general, purulent expectoration."

Whether profuse hemorrhage was more common in his day than now, we cannot affirm; but we believe such to have been the case, from the greater prevalence of inflammatory complications; and we must forget that errors in diagnosis must have then been much more frequent than now. Certainly the amount of blood which is usually lost is too small to have the least significance. Such persons are divisible into two classes, 1st. Those who believe the blood to proceed from the lungs, and to indicate mischief already commenced; and 2dly. Those who regard it as an indication of a condition of system in which phthisis will most probably occur. The determination of the site of the hemorrhage is the most important part of this inquiry.

It is presumed that the hemorrhage, when in small quantity, necessarily proceeds from the lungs, but, as we believe, without any warrant. There is no pretence of being able, by any kind of examination, to find out the site of the hemorrhage; and it is only because the blood appears with the expectoration, and both are induced by cough, and that there is a presumed connection of them with chest diseases, that that assumption has been arrived at. But when we even cursorily investigate the facts of the case, we shall admit that it is in the highest degree improbable that it could proceed from the lungs.

We have already seen that in the early stage of the disease the sputa is usually derived from the mucous surface of the pharynx and fauces; and, therefore, the fact of their being accompanied by blood, would be no evidence that the latter came from the lungs. Moreover the blood is not mixed up with each portion of the sputa, as we find in pneumonic expectoration (which, doubtless, proceeds from the structure of the lung), but is simply a streak, lying upon or within the small sputum. Its small quantity, and its appearing only on one or a very few occasions at a time, and quite apart from the sputum, renders it in the highest degree improbable that it could have been produced in the lung. Then add to these facts that it was first noticed with a somewhat severe temporary cough, and that the pharynx is often highly irritable, that enlarged and vascular follicles frequently co-exist, that enlarged veins are frequently seen upon the posterior wall of the pharynx, that specks of blood may also be seen there after severe coughing, that a violent cough so acts upon the pharynx as to render the surface quite sore—to scrape it, as patients often remark—and we are led to believe that the seat of the hæmoptysis is almost always in the pharynx in the early stage of phthisis.

It may be more difficult to discern the seat of large emissions of blood, which are sometimes said to occur. We must, however, bear in mind how certain it is that the quantity is less than it seems to be, from the discoloration of a large quantity of mucus which a small quantity of blood will effect, from the impossibility of estimating the two separately, even when carefully examined, and the natural disposition which exists to magnify an alarming occurrence, and we shall arrive at the conviction that in these cases the quantity expectorated was much less than it appeared to be. But we have seen numerous cases in which there was large and even repeated hæmoptysis, without any evidence whatever, on the most careful examination, of any destruction of the lung tissue, and in which the progress of the case during many months proved that the diagnosis was correct. In these cases also there can be no doubt that the seat of the hemorrhage was the mucous membrane either of the pharynx or of the larger bronchi, and more probably the latter. We venture to affirm that very large emissions of blood may occur in persons in the early stage of phthisis without any inflammation or marked local congestion of any part of the lungs, and be due to the rupture of a small vessel upon the mucous lining of the pharynx or larger air-tubes.

What, then, is the true significance of hæmoptysis?

1. It is not *necessarily* indicative of disease of the lung such as would imply any destruction of parts, or any local interference with the circulation in the part, as by the deposition of tubercular or other matter.

2. It most commonly indicates a state of local congestion, or increased vascularity of the pharynx, induced by numerous causes from without, in which the lungs may possibly not share, and of which they certainly are not the cause. The most common of these

causes are doubtless the temperature of the inspired air and the congestion of parts, and then the violent action of a current of air suddenly and violently rushing over a delicate surface in coughing. It is, therefore, commonly local and apart from the lungs, and due to causes acting locally.

This statement is further supported by the frequency with which hæmoptysis is met with in chronic bronchitis. We have not made a special inquiry to determine this question, but on examining the records of 3000 of our patients, we find 459 cases to which we may now refer. It is recorded that of that number, 131 had spat blood, and 155 had not spat blood; whilst in 173 cases the fact was not recorded, and hence we cannot be certain that the question was asked. This last aspect is a very common one in hospital statistics, but it nearly invalidates the whole inquiry; for we are not at liberty to infer that such cases had not spat blood. If we compare those who were recorded to have spat blood with those recorded not to have spat blood, the percentage of the former will be 45.8; but if we add the cases in which no record was made to those which are recorded not to have spat blood, the proportion of those who spat blood is reduced to 28.5 per cent.

3. There can be no doubt that the interference with the circulation which follows from lessened breath-motion of the lungs must induce a tendency to congestion, both of the pulmonary and bronchial system of vessels, and therefore so far tend, on due cause being given, to effusion of blood; but as the change in the respiration proceeds slowly, and this disturbance begins by small degrees, it is probable that in ordinary cases this is not an important cause of hæmoptysis until a later stage than that which we are now discussing. There are, however, numerous instances in which severe hæmoptysis has immediately preceded the occurrence of phthisis, and which was readily traced to local congestion of the lungs.

But whilst the foregoing may be admitted, the question is still left unanswered, "Why does hæmoptysis so frequently occur in the early stage of phthisis?" and to this we will now endeavour to give an answer.

It may be remarked that there are but few persons, however healthy, who have not had slight hæmoptysis at some period of their life—a mere streak or speck—which, at the time, they attributed to sudden cough or violent exertion; and it is no answer to say that such were probably predisposed to phthisis, and may ultimately fall into it, because the occurrence may have taken place years before, and no change in the health have since appeared.

Again, we believe that slight affections of the pharynx are far more common than has hitherto been believed; and whilst Horace Green and some other distinguished men have done much to call general attention to the diseases of the throat, they have rather led us to look for more important signs of mischief than mere irritability with congestion of vessels, and therefore have not supplied this defect.

There are few persons in whom there is not found some suffusion of the mucous membrane, and one or more enlarged vessels, if a few examinations of the pharynx be carefully made.

Further, we must recollect that phthisis is the most prevalent of all mortal diseases, and destroys one-sixth to one-eighth of the inhabitants of these islands, and far exceeds in frequency any other condition of disease.

If then we have two conditions which are very prevalent, what otherwise could occur but that both will be present together in the larger portion of cases? The marvel would be, if they did not so occur; and yet it by no means follows that there is any true dependence of the one upon the other. We hear of physicians finding scrofula or rheumatism in almost every condition of system; and since these affections are capable of considerable extension, according to the views of the individual, and are doubtless prevalent, what so certain as that they will find them in a large proportion of any cases? So, indeed, would it be with indigestion and disordered state of the bowels, which are universal, and yet not necessarily associated with, or indicative of, any particular form of disease.

But we are led by these considerations to the opinions of those who attach importance to hæmoptysis, simply, or chiefly, as indicative of a state of system in which phthisis is apt to arise, and we think that they have grounds for this belief. It is quite within belief that the local causes of hæmoptysis may be more potential in certain persons than in others, precisely as we find variation in the influence of all agencies whatever. But it is a fact, we believe, that there is a preponderance in this country of a certain form or forms of constitution in which phthisis more commonly shows itself; and as this is the prevalent kind of system, any other disease which largely prevails must appear in it also. Hence, whilst it may be true that hæmoptysis and phthisis both prevail in the community, and are both commonly found in certain forms of constitution, it does not follow that there is any connection between them, except that they may be more or less due to a common cause—a cause, however, which is subjected to much disturbance by the action of temporary influences.

CHAPTER XIX.

VOMITING.

A tendency to vomiting not unfrequently occurs.

We do not know that in the instances in which vomiting occurs there are evidences of any especial disorder of the stomach, and hence we do not think that the primary cause of it is associated with indigestion. We have already mentioned, that in many cases of early phthisis there are some evidences of dyspepsia—more frequently than is found in an equal number of persons in moderate health—and, therefore, if vomiting occur in any large number of such cases, it will be associated with dyspepsia, but we believe that usually the former is not due to the latter.

As a general rule, the vomiting or retching is due to the act of coughing, and is therefore truly pharyngeal. The cough in such cases is commonly irritable, and possibly spasmodic, and the patient continues to cough until he retches. It also not unfrequently occurs after a meal, but even then it is always associated with cough. In such cases the food excites the cough either by its quality, its presence on the pharyngeal membrane, or by the distension of the stomach preventing the usual descent of the diaphragm, and in such conditions as we have already stated there is commonly increased sensitiveness of the mucous membrane. Hence, there is a favourable conjunction of circumstances for the occurrence both of the cough and the retching, quite apart from any primary action from the stomach.

The proportion of cases in which this symptom occurs in early phthisis is but small, and is almost restricted to such as evince much sensibility of the pharynx and the general system, or who have the habit of eating quickly, or of taking too much fluid or solid food at once. It is a symptom which, in the stage now under discussion, is never permanent, but passes away in a few days. During its continuance it is, however, a symptom of urgent character, and occasionally produces much prostration of the system.

CHAPTER XX.

THE LUNGS.

THE RELATION OF THE LUNGS TO THE GENERAL SYSTEM IN PHTHISIS.

WE have now concluded our observations upon the state of the general system in the early stage of phthisis, and proceed to inquire into the condition of the organs which may be concerned or more essentially implicated in the disease in question; but, before doing so, it may be well to define the relations which exist between those two parts of the body in reference to the production of phthisis.

It is evident, as we have already shown, that the lungs must share in any change in the general condition of the system, and also that they may have their own local deviations from health, which will implicate the general system in proportion as they are more or less extensive. Hence, whether the general system suffer first, the lungs will suffer also; or whether the lungs are affected first, the system will be affected also; so that whilst any disease may be said to be local, it might with equal truth be affirmed that no disease is local. What, then, is the state of the case in reference to phthisis in its early stage?

In reference to phthisis in an advanced condition, we have no doubt as to its presenting local evidence of disease in the lungs, for the changes of structure are marked, and attract attention. In regarding the disease step by step in a yet earlier stage, we find less and less evidence of the existence of the material which is regarded as pathognomonic of phthisis, until it may be found only in a small portion of one lung, instead of its wider distribution over larger portions of one or both lungs. Having thus arrived at a point at which only the smallest amount of this recognized evidence of the disease exists, it is commonly presumed that we have found the earliest evidence of the lung disease—the commencement of the local disease; but knowing that there are conditions of the general system indicative of ill health existing even prior to this period, we transfer our attention from the lung, where the disease would be regarded as local, to the general system, and connect this state of the general system with the local conditions, not by any necessary tie, but by an accidental one, and regard the general conditions as predisposing *causes*, from which the local disease may or may not issue. Hence the general conditions of the system are regarded as only predisposing to the local mischief, and the local disease is believed to begin, not during the whole period of action of these predisposing influences, but only after a certain duration has occurred and a new substance has been deposited in the lung, which has been seized upon as the origin and essence of phthisis. So that, strictly speaking, phthisis is at no period a general disease, and as a local disease it commences only when certain morbid products *have been* deposited in the lungs.

This is, we believe, a correct statement of the belief at the present day; and it will be observed that it makes no account of the fact, that the general conditions which early occur, and which are called predisposing, are precisely those which are found through every subsequent stage of the disease, varying only in intensity; and also that the matter which has been deposited in the lung, and which marks the commencement of the local disease, must have had a source whence it was derived, and an antecedent morbid action by which it was created. How, then, can we regard a condition of the general system which exists throughout the whole course of the disease as a predisposing condition only, and in what way are we entitled to affirm that the local disease commenced in the lungs with the deposit of tubercle, when that deposit must have been due to pre-existent changes. We ask if the distinctions which have been drawn as to predisposing and local conditions are not purely arbitrary, and have arisen from the defective knowledge of former times, by which tubercular deposit was regarded as the essence of the disease, both because it was the condition of the lung readily detected, and because it having been found in some, it was affirmed to exist in all stages of phthisis? Such a view might have been the best possible one under these conditions of knowledge, but now it must be admitted that, until we have satisfied ourselves that there is not an earlier condition of disease in the lungs than that marked by the deposition of tubercle, we are not warranted in stating that tubercular deposition is the commencement of the local disease. Neither—as it is shown that there is a morbid state of the general system, which is known to precede the tubercular deposition, and which, in an unbroken line, continues throughout the course of the disease—are we entitled to dissociate this state of the general system from the local condition of the lungs, and say that the one is simply a predisposing series of events to the other. We admit the occurrence of predisposing causes and conditions on the one hand, and the deposition of tubercle as a local condition of the lung on the other; but it has been our endeavour to prove that the so-called predisposing condition is co-ordinate and alike in nature with the condition of the lung; and we now hope to show that there are conditions of the lung which precede the deposition of tubercle, and are co-existent with the change which takes place in the general system.

There has, however, been an indirect admission of the fact that tubercular deposit cannot be the first stage of the disease, and, in consequence, we find a casting about for a general condition of the system which may be proved to directly lead to the production of the tubercular matter; but nothing has yet been adduced to show why the tubercular matter, if formed at a distance from the lungs, should select those organs as its depositary, nor any tangible method by which it could be carried into them.

The part of the general system which has naturally engaged the attention of inquirers into this matter has been the blood; and as there must be different states of that fluid under many conditions, and particularly in different constitutions, it has been affirmed that there is a peculiar crasis of the blood applicable to the production of tubercular matter, and found in phthisical cases. Whilst admitting the general principles involved in this argument, we assert that there is no evidence of any known condition of the blood necessarily or even usually found in phthisis. In a course of lectures published by us in the *Association Medical Journal* for 1856, we endeavoured to controvert the statements made by Rokitansky, and must refer to them for the arguments which may be used against such a theory; but it is unnecessary to discuss the subject here at any length, since the author of the theory has withdrawn it from his subsequent editions. There is, therefore, nothing before the profession, but the general statement or belief that the origin of tubercular disease is in the blood, without any attempt to isolate the morbid product, or to define the nature of the change in that fluid from the conditions of health.

Hence, whether the statement be true or false, it is not supported by any evidence, and is mere assertion, and, at the most, a parallelism of facts. Virchow has recently drawn attention to the fact, that there is no necessary connection between the morbid action known as tuberculous and phthisis.

We do not need to offer here any remarks upon the absence of information in reference to the selection of the lungs for this deposit, since we are not aware of any attempt to explain the fact beyond the general statement, that we do not know much as to the cause of the selection of certain other organs as the depositaries of secretion; as, for example, the liver and lungs in pyæmia, and the joints in gout. The latter assertion is doubtless too true, but it cannot be the less true that there may be some special cause within the organ itself to which it is due, and which it is our duty to carefully investigate. Hitherto, no special cause in the lungs has been generally admitted, but one has been pointed out which we believe to be in the highest degree probable, and which we shall presently discuss.

As to the transmission of the diseased product to the lungs, we may remark that there are two sets of opinions upon this point—one[1] affirming that the débris of effete tissue, and the products of ill-organized nutritive matter, are deposited in the lungs, and these must of necessity have passed bodily through the capillary walls previous to their deposition. By this theory, parts of epithelial scales, tubercle cells, &c., must have not only been admitted into the blood, but have found their way out of the bloodvessels through the capillary walls. This view is very modern, but it seems to carry its own refutation so clearly with it, that we may dismiss it from the discussion with the remark, that if the blood corpuscle does not pass through capillary walls under ordinary conditions, we can scarcely expect epithelial scales and tubercle cells to penetrate them; and that if the latter could pass, it would of course follow, that the smaller blood corpuscle would pass, and that a large effusion of red blood would occur with the white tubercle.

The other one is the more philosophical one, viz., that a blastema of a morbid character is thrown out from the blood into the lungs, and after deposition takes on the cell growth, which constitutes tubercle. This blastema has not been detected, nor its characters proved.

[1] Timms on Consumption.

CHAPTER XXI.

EXTERNAL PULMONARY EVIDENCES OF PHTHISIS.

WE now proceed to discuss the conditions which are connected with the lungs in the early stage of phthisis.

LESSENED MOVEMENT OF THE CHEST.

If the observer place himself immediately in front of a patient whose chest has been uncovered, he will not fail to notice a diminution in the chest movement. The patient should sit at ease, and yet with the back tolerably erect, and with the arms hanging naturally at his side, and not resting upon any extraneous support. The ordinary mode of respiration should then be attentively watched whilst the patient is quite quiet and at his ease, and it will be noticed that the anterior and lateral elevation of the chest proceeds to a less degree than in health. This will be particularly seen in the upper and anterior parts, where the whole movement can be grasped by the eye, and where the ordinary amount of movement in health is more commonly observed and studied than at the lower part. It will also be frequently observed that there is flattening below the clavicles, and a falling in above the clavicles at the site of the apices of the lungs, although the clavicles may be in their lowest position, and not raised and fixed as in severe cases of bronchitis. It will also often occur that this flattening, or falling in, and the lessened breath movement will be less on one side than on the other, indicating generally that the progress of the disease has been greater on one side than on the other; but in forming this opinion, it will be necessary to consider the relative size of the pectoral muscles of the two sides of the chest, for they commonly differ somewhat, and in persons who employ the right arm in laborious occupations they vary considerably. It will also frequently be seen that the intercostal spaces do not exhibit their normal fulness, and particularly if the patient be thin; and although this does not usually strike the unpractised eye at first, it is occasionally so marked as to show distinct depressions.

If we now turn to the back aspect of the body, it will be seen that the motion is indistinct, so much so as to require attention to detect it with certainty. It is also common to find a little tendency to roundness of the shoulders, and also to an increase of width between scapulæ. The flatness above the transverse process of the scapulæ is also usually evident.

With these various changes it will be noticed that there is no increase in the abdominal movements, nor any unusual expansion of the thorax at its lower part.

When considering these circumstances, it will be readily understood that their due appreciation will depend upon the amount of knowledge which the observer has as to the movements and form of the chest in health—information which must include not only the average movement in all persons in health, but also the peculiarities of the individual, as to height, width of chest, and sedentary or active habits : all of which exert a material influence upon the normal amount of chest-movement. It is also requisite to recognize the broad distinction in the chest-movement, which occurs in the sexes. It is well known that in women there is usually much more breath-movement at the upper part of the chest than is found in men ; a difference due, doubtless, to the unequal pressure exerted by the stays, which constringe the lower part of the chest, but allow the upper part to act freely. Hence there may be much diminution in the chest-movement in women, and yet the amount remaining be equal to that which occurs in men ; and a reduction to the amount observed in men shows far greater diminution of breath-movement than could be inferred from an equal diminution in men. It is important, therefore, to bear in mind, that small breath motion has very different significance in the two sexes, and as it is normally so much greater in women than in men, the smaller variations are more readily recognized in the former. Hence, in studying this condition of the chest, it is better to select women than men.

To one whose eye has been well trained to appreciate minute changes in the chest-movement, no other test is required, but there are many who seek other means of admeasurement. For this purpose some place the fingers of the hand upon each shoulder, to obtain a tolerably fixed point, and then, stretching out their thumbs to various parts of the chest, attempt to measure the amount of motion. This method has but little that is rigorous in it, and would scarcely at all aid the practised eye.

The two instruments which are now commonly used for this purpose are Sibson's and Quain's chest measures, and with either of them a moderate amount of accuracy may be obtained. Sibson's instrument, consists of a metal lever, connected with a pointer and graduated dial, by the intervention of a silk thread and spring. One end of the lever is placed upon the chest, or upon the finger when laid upon the chest, and the dial being held firmly in the hand, the lever moves up and down, and varies the position of the pointer as the movements of the chest vary. It requires much practice to be able to hold the dial so firmly, that, on the one hand, no pressure shall be made by it upon the end of the lever which is in contact with the chest ; and, on the other, that the contact of the lever and the chest shall always exist; for it will readily be understood that the lever will rise and the pointer move by pressure downwards of the hand, as well as by pressure upwards of the chest; and also that, if the contact be not well sustained, there may be a degree of movement of the chest which will pass unregistered. In the hands of one well practised in its use—as, for example, in those of its inventor—we cannot doubt the accuracy of the results; but in other hands insufficiently practised, it will as certainly cause error.

But the least fallacious experimental method is that of measuring the amount of inspired air, and by this, as we have already stated, it may be proved that in the stage of disease now under discussion, there is a marked diminution in the amount of air which is inspired at each inspiration.

It is scarcely necessary to state that the amount of variation in the chest-movement, and in the form of the chest, will be proportioned to the amount of deviation from health, and therefore will vary with each person examined. We affirm that there is a diminution in the breath-movement in every case, and that as time progresses, it increases and leads to other abnormal conditions.

EXPANSIBILITY OF THE LUNGS.

The structure of the lung facilitates expiration but not inspiration.
During the expansion of the chest, the capacity of that cavity is increased in all directions at the same time, so that the lung increases in size, both in its perpendicular and transverse diameters; but, as the central part or root of the lung remains fixed, the greater portion of the expansion takes place in front of, above and below the root. The lungs are composed of two principal structures, and it must be by the expansion of one or both of these structures that its enlargement is effected. Of these two there is no evidence to show that the tubular structure has any power of elongation, although, from the arrangement of its muscular fibres, it has a power of contraction and expansion within very narrow limits around its own axis. Neither is there any evidence of any method whereby the tubular structure may be folded, so that at one time the peripheral extremity of the tube may be more distant from the central tube than at others, although this may probably occur in a small degree. There is also a small amount of movement in the lower part of the trachea and the large bronchi during the movement of the chest, but it is not in the direction of the long axis of the tube, and is only an undulating movement from behind forwards. Hence, it follows, that the whole expansion of the lung is due to the structures of those parts which lie between and at the extremities of the minute bronchial tubes, and which constitute the vesicular structure of the lungs.

Let us, therefore, ask by what mechanical arrangement this vesicular structure is enabled to expand in both uniform and diverse degrees during a long life.   The structure of these organs, as commonly described, is that of a basement membrane, having in its walls yellow elastic tissue, lying chiefly in bands, and lined on the surface with tessellated epithelium.   There is, therefore, nothing in this structure which will facilitate expansion, and the power by which the expansion is effected must be from without; in the muscles attached to the parietes of the chest, which draw the yielding structures in such directions as will enlarge the capacity of the cavity, and in this act the air enters and fills the newly created space.   The structure of the lung offers no aid whatever in this movement, but it must possess within itself a capability of being expanded, and that must be at least co-equal with the power to enlarge the cavity of the thorax from without, or an impediment to the expansion would be offered by the vesicular structure.   The capacity for expansion is therefore proportionate to the size of the vesicles above that which is required at their point of least expansion, and their ready expansibility will depend partly upon the force of the expanding power, and partly upon the amount of resistance which their own structures possess.   Hence it is seen that, whilst the structure of the lungs offers no aid in the expansion of those organs, it may offer a degree of resistance to the expansion, either by congenital or other defects, by which the capacity for expansion is unequal to the chest movement, or by varying degrees of resiliency or elasticity, by which the structures vary in the degree of opposition which they make to their expansion.

When, therefore, we find that there is a lessened degree of expansion of the chest, we may seek for its cause—without the lung, either in the degree of power by which the chest is expanded, and the expansibility of the walls of the chest; or within the lung, in the lessened capacity of the vesicles to expand, or in the increased resistance of their structures to the act of expansion.   And, further, in reference to resistance to expansion in a given time, with a certain degree of freedom, we must recollect that the tubular structure may play an important part.   The capacity of tubes to transmit fluids in a given time, varies with the square of their diameters, and therefore, with the immense number of tubular ramifications in the lungs, each one becoming smaller, there is increasing resistance to the current of the air through them, and increase of time, or of force, is required to convey the air as the tubes become smaller.   It is, therefore, a question worthy of close observation, if there is in all lungs a sufficient area in the small tubes to allow the air to pass with the required freedom under the influence of a given power, and this would be especially valuable in those cases in which there is such an impediment to respiration from birth, that it is perceptible in ordinary respiration, or at least with a small amount of exertion, and requires an inspiratory force beyond that which men ordinarily employ.   It is also now believed that the circular fibres which the small bronchial tubes possess have the power to further contract the diameter of the tubes, and thus to offer another mode (and in bronchitis an effectual mode) of resistance to the expansion of the lung.

If such, then, are actions concerned in the expansion of the lung, what are those which attend the return of the expanded lung to the volume which it normally retains in a state of rest?

It is evident that less power is usually required for expiration than for inspiration, for expiration chiefly occurs by the mere withdrawal of that force which produced the expansion, and in this act the structure of the vesicles is fitted to play an important part. This is no doubt due to the retractile power of the yellow elastic fibres, which at all times seek their normal condition at rest. These fibres are arranged in two principal directions; first, in longitudinal bands, passing from the termination of a bronchial tube to the peripheral extremity of the vesicular structure into which it leads. These bands lie near to each other, so that in a preparation of vesicular structure placed in acetic acid it often occurs that more than one band may be seen in the field at the same time with a two-third or one-quarter object-glass. There are also isolated fibres passing transversely from one band to another in a direct line, but at irregular distances; and other bands of circular fibres, which are seen to project into the interior of the intercellular passages. The latter are shown in the following figure, extracted from our lectures already quoted. On looking into the interior of any vesicle or intercellular passage, it will be seen that there is a free edge around the opening, and by lowering or raising the focus, it will be evident that this does not occupy one plane, but the circumference of a circle, with a descending plane, so that, as the focus descends, the different portions of the free edge come into focus successively, until the whole may be traced, more or less, around the circumference of the cell, and descending after the manner of a spire. This may be seen in any vesicle, but it does not follow that the spiral arrangement can be traced far in every specimen, since the section of a vesicle is much more likely to be made obliquely across the tube, or at some angle in the direction of the tube, than directly across it, and in such instances the fibres which pass round the tube would be cut across, and a number of half spires, rather than one whole turn of the spire, would be observed. The drawing (Fig. 4) was taken from a fortunate section, in which the cut at one extremity was made at right angles to the tube, and therefore embraced the whole circumference of the tube; whilst at the other extremity there was an opening by which light was admitted through the whole length of the vesicle or passage. In that section, which is the best that I ever obtained, there are five spires seen, and the continuity of the spire from the top to the bottom may be traced almost without interruption. The sketch was made from the microscopic preparation magnified 400 times; but as the drawing was a work of much complexity, the free edge only has been represented, and that appears in a rough and inartistic manner. This section was shown to Prof. Sharpey in 1855.

In the contracted state of the vesicles after expiration, it follows that there must be some arrangement whereby they occupy a less space than occurred in their state of expansion. We might suppose this arrangement to be—1st, A confused crushing of them together; 2d, A condition of intussusception, whereby the elongated extremity is drawn within the vesicle or passage; 3d, An arrangement used in telescopes, whereby several parts in the length of the passage would be retracted within those nearer to the centre; 4th, An arrangement similar to that of a spiral spring, whereby each part, from the peripheral to the central end would become folded, as when the spires of a spring press closely together.

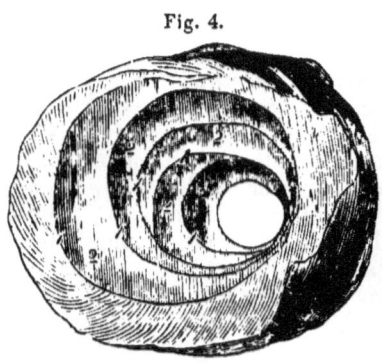

Fig. 4.

SPIRAL ARRANGEMENT OF THE AIR-CELLS.

It is clearly a condition of this folding up that the air shall be discharged from the vesicles as they contract, and that all the parts when folded shall occupy such a position that they may again be expanded with facility, or otherwise impediments both to expansion and retraction would occur. These conditions seem impossible in any arrangement by which the expanded parts should be simply crushed together, for the air would certainly be retained in the folds, and the folds would re-open with very varying degrees of facility. It is also highly improbable that these conditions would be compatible with any modification of intussusception; and, moreover, there is no arrangement of the structures which appears to indicate such an action. But the spiral arrangement to which we have drawn attention fulfils all the indications, since it admits and provides for the most orderly method of expansion and retraction, and allows the structure to be folded in the quickest manner, and to occupy the smallest space when retracted. It also requires that the air shall be removed from its peripheral extremity first, and then progressively to the central part, and permits of the most ready expansion when that act is required. When it is recollected that the alternate expansion and retraction must occur at the rate of about 1000 times per hour throughout life, and be subject to great and sudden variations of expanding force and rapidity of action, as in the case of violent exertion, it is clearly necessary that the most perfect mode of elongation and retraction should be employed. We, therefore, think that the anatomical arrangement which we have pointed out comports well with the requirements of the organ, and, in all probability, gives a sufficient explanation of this remarkable action. It may be also observed, that for this action it is not essential that the spire shall be in all its parts single, as in the bell spring, but the fibre may have a dichotomous or other arrangement, as in plants; and since the vesicles certainly communicate with each other, it is manifest that the uniformity of the spiral arrangement will be broken, in order to allow of the junction with other vesicles. In the figure above given, the spire was single and nearly uniform in its arrangement; but in the sections which will commonly occupy attention, there is much less regularity than is there depicted.

Hence, on a review of the foregoing observations, we find that the structure of the lungs in no degree aids in the expansion of these organs, yet normally passively permits the expansion whilst possessing a certain power of resistance; but it is well fitted to aid in the act of retraction. It also appears that no congenital change could confer upon it any power to aid expansion, but an abnormal arrangement might increase the natural tendency to resist expansion, and the ordinary power to effect retraction. Such also must be the effect of disease; and hence we arrive at the general conclusion that all abnormal conditions of the lungs whatever must be adverse to inspiration, and with the exception of emphysema, be favourable to expiration or both.

In the conditions met with in the early stage of phthisis, there is, as has already been shown, diminished expansion of the chest, which also implies lessened elongation, and general expansion of the air vesicles of the lung, without any diminution of the power of retraction attending expiration. It has also been shown that with this lessened amount of expansion there is also feeble inspiratory effort, and whilst the effort to expand the chest fully is less than that required to expand it to a less degree, there is a correspondence between short and feeble inspiration, and, in all probability, a more feeble motion of the air in its passage through the lungs.

CHAPTER XXII.

INTERNAL PULMONARY EVIDENCES OF EARLY PHTHISIS.
FEEBLE BREATHING.

The earliest and therefore the most universal condition is that of lessened force, and fulness of the respiratory murmur and diminished length of the ordinary inspiratory act.

Dr. Stokes remarks, in reference to feebleness of respiration, "Of the different signs of incipient phthisis there is none more important than this," and "may occur as the sole phenomenon." In giving three causes for its production, he believes with M. Reynaud that it is commonly due to obliteration of the minute bronchial tubes.

He, however, still associates it with deposition of tubercle; and it is probable from his definition of the cause of it, that he does not mean the same thing as that referred to by us. It is not necessary that there should be an irregular kind of respiration, such as would be perceived by the ear, if some of the air vesicles were pervious and others closed, as after the deposition of tubercle, but an uniform feebleness of the sound issuing from all the air vesicles equally. The condition referred to by Dr. Stokes refers, we think, to a later period.

We believe it to be a universal condition in the earliest stage of phthisis that the vesicular murmur is less strong than occurs in health. The examination may be conducted by testing both ordinary and forced inspiration. On the patient being quietly seated, and the respiration proceeding naturally, it will be found that the vesicular murmur is but indistinctly audible, and quite different from that general gentle buzzing which is so perceptibly present in health. At the same time it will be noticed that the apparent distance to which the inspired air is carried, or, in other words, the length of the inspiratory current, is shortened, and the act of inspiration is short and feeble, whilst that of expiration is perhaps shorter and quicker than is natural. On the patient inspiring forcibly the respiratory sounds are of course increased considerably in intensity, but they are more or less tubular, and the vesicular sound is much less distinct than occurs with forced inspiration in health, and there is still the same evidence of feebleness of inspiration. It also frequently occurs that the patient is unable to take a long, deep, and slow inspiration, until his attention has been repeatedly called to it, and he has been in some degree trained. Usually, when he is required to inspire deeply, he makes a quick and short inspiration, and when he has overcome that source of error, the inspiration will still be feeble, and only with difficulty can he be induced to inspire deeply, and to fully expand the lungs.

It usually occurs that whilst feeble and short vesicular sounds are extensively present, they are more perceptible on one side than on the other (Dr. Stokes and others affirm that the vesicular murmur is naturally more feeble on the right side), for it very rarely happens that the disease proceeds at an equal pace in all parts of the chest, and as the disease advances to a certain point the vesicular sounds progressively diminish in force and fulness.

It may here be demanded in what respect this change varies from that found in ordinary debility on the one hand, and from a tubercular condition on the other, and we will endeavour to answer these questions. In ordinary cases of debility there is no doubt feeble breath-motion, as there is feebleness of every other vital act, and there are also many healthy persons in whom the breath-motion and breath sounds are less strong than is found in the majority of cases. Yet, to an ear well trained to this inquiry, there is no difficulty in the diagnosis, for the degree of feebleness is far less than is found in that stage which immediately precedes tubercle, and *in all cases of mere debility the vesicular sounds and the trajet of the air become normal in deep inspirations.* This latter we hold to be the true diagnostic sign; and although the state of the ordinary respiration is often a sufficient guide, it is better for every observer, whether peculiarly trained or otherwise, to examine the condition in forced inspiration also. In practising the latter examination, it is highly important that the inspirations be not made in a rapid and jerking manner, but with ease, regularity, and moderate force, for in all conditions of the lungs in which the inspiratory effort is very forcible and rapid the tubular sounds predominate over the vesicular.

But as the general evidences of early phthisis are chiefly those of continued debility, it is evident that in states of chronic debility, from whatever cause, the chest should be frequently examined, and the progress in the diminution of the breath-sounds and chest-movements carefully ascertained; for, as the cases of phthisis number one-eighth of all our patients afflicted with fatal diseases, it follows that the states of debility leading to phthisis will be most abundant, and form a large proportion of cases of debility from all combined causes.

PROLONGED BREATH CURRENT.

The earliest evidence of the deposition of tubercle is that which indicates a localized and isolated obstruction to the current of the air.

There can be no doubt, from the structure of the lungs, that as these organs are expanded by the entering current of air, they always offer an obstruction to its entrance; but this is general, and the degree of it is included in the perception of the respiratory sounds and movements which we learn as constituting health. It can scarcely be said that this degree of obstruction is increased in the earliest stage of phthisis, for the defect is then rather in the inspiratory power than in the expansibility of the lung. Yet it is quite possible that as the disease advances to the period when tubercle is deposited, and particularly if the progress be slow, the expansibility of the lung will diminish in proportion to the lessened expansion, and increased obstruction will be offered to the entrance of the air. But whilst this may be so theoretically, we do not find in practice any sign by which its existence may be distinguished from the mere diminution of inspiratory power or effort.

When, however, a foreign body of an appreciable bulk is deposited within the air cells, and lessens their capacity, it is evident that in its degree it lessens or prevents the entrance of air into, and the expansibility of, the particular vesicles. In this condition, it is clear that there is increased obstruction to respiration, and the earliest indications of the deposition will be the evidences of the obstruction. The obstruction will be opposed both to the ingress

and egress of air.   There must be a period when the first alone is
present, since it occurs within the air vesicles affected, but practically
after a period both occur together.   After a few vesicles have become
partially filled with the deposit, they press upon the adjoining ter-
minal branches of the bronchial tubes, or of the air passages leading
to other air vesicles, and become an accumulating cause of the closure
of the air vesicles.   In the earliest condition the signs are those of
further diminution of vesicular expansion, and, consequently, greater
prominence of tubular breathing, and these may continue for an indefinite period ; but when the second condition above mentioned
occurs, the impediment to breathing may be particularly shown by
the prolonged respiration, or a lagging behind in the current of air
at the parts affected.   This, doubtless, occurs in both the inspiratory
and expiratory acts, but chiefly in the latter ; and it is at least in
part due to the fact, that as the volume of air in the vesicles beyond
the obstruction is small, and can only be forced out by pressure conducted from the parietes of the chest to the more deeply seated parts
of the lungs, it cannot overcome the resistance with the same rapidity and force as occurs in inspiration, when the volume of the air
behind it is large, the muscular effort greater, and the force is applied to that particular current in a more direct manner.   Hence,
the obstruction is more easily overcome by inspiration, and any
sound which it might produce is lost in the louder tubular sounds,
and is soon checked by the immediately succeeding act of expiration ;
whilst in expiration the power is more feeble and less direct, and
the interval of rest following the act of expiration allows much time,
during which the air may continue to pass outwards, and the sounds
of expiration be heard.

WAVY OR JERKING RESPIRATION.

We do not think that wavy or jerking respiration is evidence of
the deposition of tubercle or of any other material, nor, indeed, essentially of any obstruction within the lungs, but at the same time
its presence in early phthisis deserves attention.   We have seen
numerous instances, and particularly in persons who breathe feebly,
in which it has evidently resulted from an irregular mode of breathing, and was connected directly or indirectly with muscular action.
In a few cases we have found this sign present in every part of the
lungs ; but usually it is more restricted in extent.   In many others
we have found it in cases of chronic bronchitis, without any evidence
whatever of deposition, but with much obstruction to the current of
air.   In a third class we have found it associated with tubercular
deposition in every stage of the disease, except that it was not heard
in the parts of the lungs in which the process of excavation was present.   Hence, we believe it to occur under two perfectly distinct
sets of conditions, in only one of which is there obstruction within
the lungs to the entrance of air, and in that it may be due to con-

traction of the air tubes, whether of a bronchitic or tubercular kind. The conditions under which we think its presence of value, as indicating the presence of tubercle, is where there is an absence of bronchitic contraction and irregular breathing, and where it is localized in a space of one or two inches, and passes away as the deposit increases. Hence, whilst we would attach value to this sign when conjoined with others of a more trustworthy character, we do not, upon the whole, think that its presence or absence is of much importance in the diagnosis of this particular disease.

DULNESS ON PERCUSSION.

Dulness on percussion is a sign of great importance, but it occurs in very different degrees and under very different conditions.

It is impossible for two persons to arrive at the same idea of the value of this sign, unless they are in the habit of attaching the same value to degrees of dulness, and of eliciting the sound in the same manner. There are many who do not recognize the fitness of the term until the degree is so considerable that it may be readily recognized at a distance from the patient, and who elicit the same by violent thumps of the ends of several fingers, or the knuckles, or by a hammer. Such cannot be expected to recognize those lesser degrees which require the ear to be brought near to the patient, and the most sensitive of the two ears to be directed to the side percussed, nor such sounds as are elicited by a quick and smart, but not heavy blow, by the index finger upon the back of a finger of the other hand well pressed upon the chest. There can be no doubt that in most cases, both light and heavy percussion should be made, but we maintain that it is impossible to appreciate minute changes without the gentle yet firm kind of percussion, an ear quick at the perception of sound, the direction of the ear to the chest, and the earnest attention of the mind to the inquiry. Hence, with all these necessary conditions, it is very manifest that many will never be able to appreciate the minute changes, and that others will confound all the degrees of dulness under the marked expression of that sign.

But to these we must further add the natural variations of sound on percussion in healthy persons, due no doubt in large measure to the thickness of the chest parietes, and to the age of the patient, and not yet fully explained. Other things being equal, the sound on percussion is much clearer in the young than in the old, and in spare than in fat and muscular persons, and as this must be duly allowed for, and yet its degree be not capable of absolute determination, it will under all circumstances be a small source of error. As a general expression, we may state that the examiner with the most delicate sense of hearing, the power of abstracting his attention, and the greatest practice both in health and disease, carried on in a careful

manner, is the most likely to appreciate the earliest deviation from
health in reference to percussion and other auscultatory phenomena.

In the early stage of phthisis, before there is any evidence of the
deposition of tubercle, there is an appreciable degree of dulness on
the clavicles, and, indeed, over the chest in general.   This is not
found in the earliest condition, but only after the diminution in the
expansion of the lung has been long continued.   It arises no doubt
from the absence of the full amount of air in the lung tissue, which
was common in health, for in such cases we cannot doubt for a
moment that the solid tissues bear a larger proportion to the volume
of the lung than occurs when the air vesicles are usually expanded.
Some may think this to be over-refinement, and question its truthfulness; but let such examine the percussion note of the clavicles in
old cases of bronchitis, and the doubt will be removed, for no one
believes that in such cases there is the deposition of solid matter in
the lungs, or any large accumulation of blood there in the absence
of the winter increase of dyspnœa, and yet the percussion note is
duller than is found in conditions of phthisis far more advanced than
those now under consideration.   There is also in long-continued bronchitis a state of collapse of the apices of the lungs, as is evident by
the depression which is found above each clavicle even when the
arms are pulled down; and without entering into the question as to
the precise causes of this, we may remark that the fact is commonly
the same in old people.

The degree of dulness observed in the absence of the evidences of
tubercular deposition, varies and increases as the disease is prolonged,
and whilst it may be equally present on both sides, it more commonly
preponderates on one side.   Hence, up to this point, and without
the evidence of impeded respiration, dulness on percussion is not
evidence of the existence of tubercle.   When the deposition of tubercle begins, there is a more permanent and evident cause of dulness;
but if it proceed slowly and be greatly limited in extent, the addition
to the degree of dulness is not considerable.   The form of deposition
in which the dulness is the most pronounced, is that in which the deposit is widely distributed, and increases with moderate rapidity.
Speaking generally, as the deposit increases in each cell, and in the
mass of the cells from the surface to the more remote parts, so will
the dulness also increase; yet there is so much diversity in the degree of dulness found with tubercular deposit that the amount of deposit can be inferred in only a general manner, from the degree and
extent of the dulness alone.

SUMMARY.

Having thus considered the evidences which the external examination of the lungs furnishes in reference to phthisis, we think it may
be convenient to sum up in a few words the truths which they
represent.

1. When there is less breath-motion, less length of inspiration, and feeble yet tolerably even vesicular sounds, both with ordinary and forced respiration over the whole chest, or particularly at one or both apices, with or without slight dulness on gentle percussion of the clavicles, and without rales or any sign of bronchitis, we believe that there is the early or the pre-tubercular stage of phthisis.

2. When there is dulness at least moderately pronounced and localized, and prolonged expiration with, but sometimes without, flattening of the chest at the part affected, and with or without wavy or jerking respiration, and with unevenness of the respiratory sounds at the part affected, in addition to the signs of the first stage, and still without rales or other evidences of bronchitis, we consider that tubercle is deposited, and the disease in that part has passed into the second stage.

3. When general bronchitis is also present, the diagnosis from the examination of the chest is almost impossible, and whilst the progress of the general symptoms may aid us, a correct opinion can only be formed after the signs of old bronchitis have disappeared, or the general evidences of phthisis both in the lungs and system have increased.

4. The state of the general system is substantially the same, whether before or soon after the first deposition of tubercle, but the degree of variation from health will have increased in the latter with lapse of time. Hence, whilst this state must be considered in forming our diagnosis of phthisis, it is equally indicative in the two stages, except perhaps in degree.

CHAPTER XXIII.

PATHOLOGY OF THE FIRST STAGE OF PHTHISIS AND OF TUBERCLE.

WE now proceed to consider the evidences of the disease which are found in an internal examination of the lungs up to the limits of the period embraced by this work.

The only parts to which inquiry has hitherto been directed are the minute divisions of the bronchial tubes and the air cells. The distribution of the bloodvessels has also been examined—not with a view to show any connection between them and the occurrence of the disease, but to ascertain whether they penetrate the tubercular masses, and to what extent they remain pervious.

We have already shown that the structure of the minutest bronchial tubes is quite different from that of the air cells, since the former consists of a series of coats of various structures, lined by ciliated epithelium, and, so far as is known, varying little in length

6

during the acts of respiration, whilst the latter have a basement membrane, with a delicate tessellated epithelium on the inner, and bands of yellow elastic tissue on the outer surface, and submit to elongation and retraction with every act of respiration. Hence there is a *primâ facie* objection to any identity of diseases to which they may be subject, and the former will more commonly exhibit diseases allied to those of mucous, and the latter to those of serous surfaces.

The universal belief of the present day is, that the bronchial tubes are not primarily concerned in the disease in question, and that they become implicated by extension of diseased products outwards from the air vesicles, or from the pressure of lateral masses. In the former case they can only be regarded as depositories or, as it may be, channels of transit of diseased products elsewhere generated, whilst, in the latter, they may seriously add to the mischief by interfering with the ingress of air to the vesicles to which they lead, and thus cut off portions of the lung from the performance of their functions.

Hence, we turn primarily to the air vesicles of the lung, with a view to ascertain in what manner these organs exhibit evidences of phthisis.

FIRST STAGE.

There have not as yet been any inquiries made as to the state of the air vesicles in the stage preceding that of deposit, and, indeed, such would, in the present state of science, be nugatory, for so long as there is a difference of opinion as to the existence of a layer of epithelium, and the normal arrangement and structure of the air cells is matter of dispute, it is impossible to educe anything in reference to their minute changes in disease which shall be worthy of attention. Hence, those who oppose the view of a precursory pre-tubercular stage have the advantage of this negative evidence.

But satisfactory and complete evidence is not attainable in inquiries into any vital action until those inquiries have been long continued; and, in the mean time, it is permitted to adduce such presumptive evidence as the existing state of knowledge affords.

It is an established law in the animal economy that a structure retains its full healthy vitality when in the full performance of its functions, and that, *cæteris paribus*, it tends to disease whenever these actions are unduly increased or decreased. This is well established in reference to the action of the heart, the muscles of the limbs, and the functions of the liver and brain, as indeed of every organ and tissue in the body. Hence, as we have shown that in cases of early phthisis the actions of the lungs, both physical and vital, are diminished, and that commonly this diminution has been long continued, we must admit that they are brought into a condition removed from the standard of health, and have become more liable to put on the marks of disease, and, in accordance with their conformation, to become the depositories of diseased products. We cannot think that any one can raise a valid objection to the statement thus made; and we may further add, that as the tissues of the lungs are a part of the general tissues of the body, and the nutrition of the lungs must be supplied from the same source as the nutrition of the general system, it follows, that with a state of the general system, in which the evidences of lessened vitality exist, there will be a corresponding state of the lungs themselves. Dr. C. Radclyffe Hall, in his interesting little work on Torquay, when discussing the nature of consumption, remarks: "But in order for tubercle to form in the first instance, the portion of lung about to be affected must be in an unhealthy condition, to begin with; and the blood brought to it must be unhealthy. The earliest local deviation from health in the lung I believe to consist in an atrophy of the delicate filmy tissue which lines the walls of the air-cells. This atrophy depends upon a diminution in the vital power of nutrition in the part." Hence, we venture to assert that in the early stage of phthisis, before the deposition of tubercle, there is a condition of lessened vitality of the air vesicles of the lungs, and an unusual tendency to the reception of morbid matters.

The chronological relation of this condition to the other evidences of the disease may be variously regarded. There can be no doubt that such a condition, however induced, is well fitted to lessen still further the degree of vital action of the tissues, and thereby to become an efficient cause in the progress of the disease, but it can scarcely be regarded as the cause of co-existent conditions, since we have assumed, that, in a majority of cases at least, there was a period when the vital actions were performed in the lungs in a manner consistent with health; and we must therefore look to an anterior cause, or that upon which the healthy state depends, to find the reason for this departure from the healthy state. We have shown that the step immediately preceding this is lessened action of the lungs, and this must be due to the muscular power by which the action is maintained, to the vital changes in the tissues, which, as has been shown by Dr. Flint,[1] are the cause of the *besoin de respirer*, and finally to that power upon which all vital action primarily depends. Without being able to penetrate into the latter,

[1] "American Medical Journal," Oct. 1861. The conclusions to which Dr. Flint's interesting investigations led him are as follows:—

"1. That the *besoin de respirer* does not occur during the continuance of artificial respiration. 2. It is felt when respiration is impeded or arrested. 3. Also when the blood becomes black; and 4. During the emission of blood, and whilst artificial respiration is maintained, the *besoin de respirer* occurs after a certain quantity of blood has been lost and before general convulsions supervene."

Hence he infers that it is due to the want of oxygen in the tissues, and as an inference we may remark that it will be the less felt in proportion to the less degree of vital action in the tissues, and consequently in early phthisis.

we have shown that the two preceding conditions exist in phthisis, but in the present state of our knowledge we cannot demonstrate such a sequence in the order of events as to show clearly the period when the condition of the general system had the immediate precedence of that of the lungs. There can be no doubt, however, upon the same reasoning, that as in different persons the degree of health, or of vital resistance, differs from their birth, those who inherit or receive at their birth a system deficient in vital power, are more prone to this condition of the lungs than others having a more vigorous state of health.

SECOND STAGE—TUBERCLE.

We next proceed to consider the evidences of phthisis after tubercle has been deposited.

In our historical sketch at p. 29, we have given the outlines of the opinions which were held by Baillie, Bayle, Laennec, and Carswell, in reference to the appearance of tubercle in its various stages, and shall only now refer to such statements as may be found in the works of the two latter authors. Laennec refers to seven forms of tubercle, arranged under the two heads of insulated and infiltrated matter.

Of the insulated forms the *Miliary* tubercle is the most common, and resembles small grains which are gray and semi-transparent, sometimes even transparent and colourless. They grow in distinct bodies, but after a period they increase and approach each other, and form groups. There is a yellow speck observed in the centre, or, as Andral affirms, in other parts of each tubercle, and ultimately the whole body becomes yellow; and as at that period the group of tubercles has become one homogeneous body of a whitish yellowish colour, they require another designation, that of *Crude* tubercle. The *Granular* tubercle of Bayle is very rare, and is distinguished from the foregoing by the fact, that the small millet-seed-sized granules always remain distinct, and are transparent or semi-transparent, and colourless or slightly gray. In the infiltrated forms of tubercle, the whole of the part of the lung in which they occur appears to be equally occupied by the matter, as, for example, the parts around vomicæ, and in the interstices of the groups of miliary tubercle, and after a variable period it consists of tubercular matter, mingled with pus and other fluids, the result of secondary changes. In some instances, therefore, this matter will appear as a gray and consistent substance, and then it is termed *gray infiltration*, whilst in others it assumes a gelatinous form, and in a third class it is evidently purulent. In the opinion of Laennec and his contemporaries, tubercle of every kind is first gray and semi-transparent, and the yellow character is due to subsequent changes, but Carswell controverted that statement, and affirmed that the former does not necessarily precede the latter. The former commonly appears in the air cells and on serous membranes. Rokitansky has varied the nomenclature of these different conditions, but it is not necessary to refer here to his excellent work.

We shall not quote the opinions of Baillie, Bayle, and Laennec, as to the precise seat of the tubercle, for they had not the advantage of the microscopic knowledge of our day, but we simply state that they believed it to be in the cellular tissue—a term used then in a less precise and restricted sense than now. Carswell, with greater advantages, found it upon the surface of tissues, and particularly of those of hollow organs. Neither shall we enter minutely into the question of the site of the commencement of softening of tubercle, but may state that Laennec and his contemporaries believed it to begin at the centre of each mass in connection with a bloodvessel which they affirmed to be present there, whilst Carswell affirmed that the softening begins at the circumference, and that there only is there commonly a connection with the vascular system. Rainey affirms that the softening begins at the centre, because it is the furthest removed from the bloodvessels, and Rokitansky's description of the process shows it to be physical in its nature, and due to absorption of fluid from the adjoining parts. Lebert is of opinion that softening occurs both from the circumference and the centre in different instances.

Such, then is a brief outline of the appearance of tubercle to the naked eye and the changes which it undergoes, and in a few words it may be stated that tubercle commonly begins at a point and increases in quantity until it is as large as a small seed. This occurs in many places about the same time, and at length the small rounded or slightly angular bodies are pressed together until a mass is formed. The deposit is at first transparent and colourless or slightly gray, but it subsequently solidifies somewhat and becomes opaque, and finally by various stages liquefies and is expectorated from a part in process of evacuation.

We will now adduce the information which the microscope has enabled us to obtain, and trace the changes somewhat more minutely.

The material in its earliest form consists of a number of cells, varying in size, but commonly smaller than a mucous cell, filled with granules, and also a quantity of free granular matter and other non-cellular elements. At a later period the cellular element is less abundant than the granular, and pus cells and débris of tissues appear in the softened mass. The chemical composition shows the presence of an albuminous material and mineral matter.

These substances are deposited on the free surface of the air cells (but some affirm that they are also found in the parenchyma of the lung, and in the minute bronchial tubes), and in each lobule the deposit may proceed in several cells at the same time, until the further extension of the cells is hindered by the inelastic lobular membrane which incloses a number of them. In progress of time the deposit having occurred in a number of lobules, the cells of adjoining lobules become filled up, and the two masses lie in close approximation, or it may be that the adjoining lobule remains free, and then the masses remain disconnected and projecting.

Rainey has expressed our view when he says that the tubercle being deposited on the inner surface of the air cell, the latter becomes distended, and after a time the cell walls or the septa between two masses of tubercle become compressed and the intervening bloodvessels obliterated. Every tubercle may, therefore, be regarded as an air cell full of tuberculous matter, and the amount of vital action remaining in the cells will be in great part proportionate to the extent to which the bloodvessels lying outside the cell and between adjoining cells remain patent. Hence the coloured spot often used in the centre of a miliary tubercle does not, as Mr. Ancell intimates, represent the remains of the contents of the air cell, but the central point of the mass which fills the distended (not compressed) air cells.

As each air cell receives the deposit, its cavity and capability of expansion is by so much lessened, and after a period the air is admitted only to the end of the bronchial tube, unless in the mean time the lobules on the sides of the bronchial tube have compressed the tube and prevented the ingress of air to the cells to which it is directed. Hence with deposition there will be solidification and immobility of the lung, and the chief causes of variation are the extent of deposition at first, the rapidity of the filling of the individual cells and of the implication of other cells in the morbid process. Commonly a few cells or lobules are selected at first, and these are usually found in one of the apices of the lungs.

NATURE OF TUBERCLE.

Let us now ask what is the true nature and source of tubercle in the lungs? It is necessary to limit our observations to the deposit found in the lungs only, for with that alone are we concerned; and although masses of matter similar in appearance are found elsewhere, and are called tubercle, it is not certain that their nature is identical with that of those found in the lungs.

CELLULAR CHARACTER OF TUBERCLE.

The precise nature of the histological elements which are found in tubercular masses is not yet settled. They have been described as rounded or oval granular cells, but these characters are not such as would enable any histologist to determine the nature of tubercle if examined alone and apart from the other histological evidences of the mass.

The precise nature of the free granular matter, and of the various non-cellular elements which are found in tubercular masses, is at present a subject of speculation, but there is a presumption that the granular matter is derived from the cells after the cell wall has become ruptured, and that the débris may in part be the ruptured cell wall.

BLOOD ORIGIN OF TUBERCLE.

It is commonly held that the morbid material is derived from the blood. It is deposited in the amorphous form common to all deposits, but subsequently undergoes the vital transformation necessary to the formation of cells, and differs from benign deposits in having its vital development arrested at this first step of cellular growth. Hence it is deficient in plastic qualities, and instead of being convertible into some of the tissues of the body, it remains as a foreign body, and has a marked tendency to degenerate and decay. It is also affirmed that the relation between the deposition in the bronchial and other glands is such that, as in Professor Allison's case, the matter may be determined to the glands, and thus be averted from the lungs, or, as is believed by Dr. J. C. B. Williams, the tubercular matter may be removed from the lungs and deposited in the glands. In considering this blood theory, we require reasons for the following :—

1. *Why the lungs should be selected for this deposition in so vast a majority of cases.* There is nothing known in their structure which will account for it, and if it be referred to their great vascularity, we may reply that tubercle is much less frequently found in so highly vascular an organ as the liver, and is met with on serous and mucous surfaces where the vascularity is not greater than that of other tissues.

2. *The depravity of the vital processes by which this matter is produced, and which is chiefly discernible in this deposit only, if we compare its frequency with that of any other due to chronic conditions.* It is arguing in a circle to say, that because the system is not in good health, the deposits will be unhealthy, and that the deposits must be depraved because the system is unhealthy. If the depravity be due to the state of the health, then all deposits occurring in such a state should be depraved ; but this is not strictly true, for, in reference to inflammatory deposits, their nature is in great part determined by the activity of the local morbid process, which is only in a general manner influenced by the general system ; and if a matter should be regarded as depraved and unhealthy because the disease associated with it tends to death, the term can have no special significance beyond the expression of the condition of the general system, and thus we are brought back in the circle to the

proof of the connection of this deposit with the state of the general system. There can be no doubt that in early phthisis the vital transformations are not so perfect as in health. There can be no doubt also, that as the circulating medium varies in its composition according to the nutritive material taken into the system, the perfection of the acts of transformation, and the amount and nature of the effete matters removed from the tissues, it must vary in every person hourly, and in every variety of constitution, and in every disease; but it is evident that we gain no increase of knowledge by a reference to this state, unless we can point out the precise changes which have occurred, the conditions to which they are due, and the evils to which they tend. Whilst admitting the fact, we venture to state that expressions respecting it are made loosely, and without any precise idea, and in illustration we may cite the case of an American critic who, in discussing most ably the merits of Dr. Lawson's work.[1] objects to the statement that there is a stage of phthisis before tubercle is deposited, and remarks: " Before the deposit of tubercle reveals itself by physical signs, the health must be deranged, for these signs are indicative only of a certain accumulation of morbid matter." In this it will be observed that there is an explanation based upon a gratuitous assumption, for he had not proved the accumulation to exist, but assumed that because tubercle would be deposited, it must accumulate in the blood previously.

3. *The fact that the amorphous condition of the effusion has never been seen in phthisis, but, on the contrary, that in the earliest stage, and in the most newly-formed tubercle, the cell structures are present.* This statement that tubercle is deposited in an amorphous state is based upon the assumption, that because in certain other conditions an amorphous lymph is first effused, and cell-formation is set up subsequently, it therefore occurs also in this instance ; but setting aside the *non sequitur* of the argument, it is to be observed that such a statement at once begs the question by assuming that it is a deposition from the blood.

4 *The sudden arrest of that vital action which had been set up in the amorphous deposit, by which cell or nucleus growths have arisen, leaving the material as inactive or dead as if it were unorganized.*

5. *The fact that cells of the size of the tubercle cells cannot pass through the tissues, and if the cells have been disintegrated, and the matter absorbed in its granular and amorphous state, how it is accounted for that in the glands, whither it has been carried, it again appears organized.*

6. *The almost entire immunity of early youth from this disease, and the comparative infrequency of it at and after middle life.* If it be derived from a depraved state of the blood, why is it not distributed over all ages with some approach to uniformity, for at all

---

[1] The American Medical Journal, July, 1861, p. 157.

periods, and particularly in childhood, we find abundant evidence of continued ill health, and innumerable instances in which ill-formed lymph is thrown out on serous surfaces, and in external wounds ?

EPITHELIAL ORIGIN OF TUBERCLE.

Another theory has been propounded, which has the merit of simplicity and of avoiding many of the difficulties which beset the blood theory. Shrœder Van der Kolk, Addison, and many others have pointed out the resemblance which exists between the enlarged nucleus of the lung-epithelium and the cells of tubercle, and have affirmed that the tubercle is effete and accumulated epithelium of the air vesicle.

Dr. J. H. Bennett, who strongly advocates the blood theory, confesses that the tubercle cell is really a nucleus, but without a tendency to form cells. *Rokitansky* asserts that nuclei are normally present, and *Lebert* affirms that they rarely appear. *Gulliver* and *Vogel* believe that at the early period nucleated cells are formed in the tubercle, and *Virchow* asserts that tubercle originates in the interior of epithelial or other cells.

Our esteemed colleague, *Dr. Walshe,* in referring to this important statement of Virchow, somewhat ridicules such revelations of science, and thinks it better to trust to that which is evident to the eye and to ordinary observation, than to such vague results of histological science : but we mistake greatly if Professor Virchow's views do not lend valuable aid to a theory opposed to that adopted by Dr. Walshe, and probably to be preferred to it, and if it be not a true advance of knowledge. Whether the tubercle cell be due to a retrograde metamorphosis or not is a question of theory ; but that it resembles the nucleus of the epithelium cells, with which it is almost invariably found, is, we believe, a matter of fact ; and, further, it is highly probable that the tubercle is derived from the epithelium.

In this theory we find a ready explanation of the selection of the lungs for the deposit (for the material is naturally found in the place where the deposit occurs) ; of the accumulation of the deposit (from the peculiar construction of that part of the lungs, namely, a large and expanded *cul-de-sac,* in which the deposit occurs, having for its outlet a minute cone-shaped tube, the narrow end of which terminates in a *cul-de-sac*) ; of the origin of the granular cells (without supposing the setting up and arrest of a vital process in a homogeneous mass effused from the blood, which has never been demonstrated) ; of the infrequency of it in childhood (when the respiratory function is very active, and the air vesicles immature) ; of the origin of the *débris* (from the expanded part of the tubercle cell) ; and of the wide dissemination of the matter (from the universality of the same conditions). It would still remain to show why the epithelium should accumulate in disease and not in health, but that offers no serious objection to the theory, for it is fully believed that everywhere epithelium is subjected to constant degradation and renewal; and it would almost certainly follow that the air-cells, having been long inefficiently expanded, and the current of air introduced and emitted with less force, there would be parts of the unfolded cells in which the material might lodge, and the *débris* would be less easily carried into the bronchial tube. Then if we add to these facts the lessened vitality of the structures consequent upon the more feeble performance of their functions, we have the conditions fitted for the production of an epithelium of changed organization.

According to the testimony of all observers, there is but small evidence of mineral deposition in the tubercle so long as it remains transparent and colourless, and it is only in the secondary changes, which produce discoloration and opacity, that it abounds. This would comport as well with this as with the theory of the blood origin of the deposit. It would also readily account for the now established fact, that *tubercle is almost exclusively found on the surface of membranes possessing an epithelial covering*, and not in the substance of tissues, where the bloodvessels for the most part abound; and if it leave unaccounted for the source of the deposit in bones and other places where there is no epithelium, we may well admit that an erroneous opinion may exist as to the identity of the deposits when such exceptional cases bear no proportion to the number of those in which the deposit is found with epithelium.

This view appears to us to have much to commend it in a positive sense, and also negatively, by excluding the difficulties which attend the consideration of the blood theory. It also comports well with our view of the first stage of phthisis, and the manner in which the first leads to the second stage.

It is well known that the earliest seat of tubercle in the lungs is almost invariably at the apex, and so constant and singular a fact must be due to conditions especially found in that locality. On examining the apex, with a view to explain this peculiarity, we do not find anything in the intimate structure in which that differs from any other part of the lung; but in considering its function, there is something which has engaged the attention of numerous observers, and, amongst them, of Sir Robert Carswell. This acute physician remarked that tubercle is rarely found in moving organs, whilst it is so abundant in the parts of the lungs—the apices—in which there is much less motion than is found in other parts of the same organ. Hence he associates this liability to the deposition of tubercle with the small motion of the part; and it is singular to notice how well this view supports the opinions recorded in the last paragraph as to the origin of the tubercle; for if lessened breath motion lead to the deposition of tubercle, it will follow that the parts of the lungs in which the breath motion is very small in health, will be the first to put on evidences of this disease. It well accords with the view that tubercle is accumulated and transformed epithelium; but we have no explanation whatever of the reason for the selection of these parts of the lungs if the tubercular matter be deposited from the blood. In our Lectures, already referred to, we pointed out another fact which corresponds with the statement made by Sir Robert Carswell—viz., that, from the direction of the bronchial tubes and the inspiratory force, the current of air is chiefly directed to the base of the lung, and that it is only on the deepest inspiration, and when the base has become full of air, that the apices can be completely distended. This is evident on the mere inspection of the lung, but is demonstrated when either the observer attentively examines his own inspiration or that of any other person. The lessened degree of expansion, and, to a certain extent, the lessened movement of the apices, may thus be accounted for.

CHAPTER XXIV.

PROGRESS OF TUBERCLE.

It now remains to show in what manner the tubercle deposited in the lung comports itself when the tendency of the disease is towards death and towards recovery.

We have elsewhere stated that tubercle does not extend by a process analogous to the extension of cancerous deposits, viz., by infiltration and destruction of the surrounding tissues, but simply by accumulation of the same material in hollow cavities lined by the epithelial cells. Hence, the tubercle already deposited is in no degree an active vital agent, but must be regarded as a foreign body, having its own tendency to decay, and also tending to the decay of the parts in which it is placed—the latter action not, however, by any malignant virtue which it possesses, but by excluding the supply of blood to the parts and interfering with the vital functions of the organs.

Hence, up to a certain point we have simply accumulation of material, interference with the functions of the part, and lessening of the vital properties of the containing tissues.

AS TO THE TISSUES.

The changes which proceed in the tissues may be the most readily explained, and we will, therefore, first describe them. The supply of blood being cut off more or less perfectly, and the functional activities of the tissues being more or less arrested, it follows that the nutrition of the tissues will be diminished, and there will be a constant tendency to decay. This decay is evinced in two ways: 1st. By a shrivelling of the tissues as the fluid which they contain becomes more and more removed. This is observed in cases of isolated tubercle, in which calcareous degeneration has proceeded, and to which we shall again refer. 2d. By destructive disintegration. This process has been almost universally regarded as inflammatory, both from the fact that in other tissues destructive action is for the most part inflammatory, and because pus cells are found in the course of the destruction. This is a subject which is, perhaps, incapable of such investigation as may decide the question; but when we recollect, on the one hand, that the tissues involved are simply composed of a basement membrane and a number of closed capillary vessels, it is not easy to see how true inflammatory action could be set up; and, on the other, that in true inflammatory action there is commonly a blastema effused, in which organizing elements are produced, neither of which is necessarily found in this process; and, therefore, it is scarcely credible that this should be the process of disintegration in the mass of cases. Moreover, in the action in question there is no such tendency to spread rapidly as is found in ordinary pneumonia; neither does the general system show evidences of inflammatory action proceeding in a vital organ. Hence, whilst we do not deny that in some instances, and those particularly in which the tubercular masses are not closely compacted together, true inflammatory action may occur, and induce the softening of the tubercular masses; we believe that in the ordinary instances of the softening of tubercle the disintegration of the tissue proceeds chiefly by the absence of nutrition, and not by the action known as true inflammation; nay, we venture to assert, that commonly inflammation does not occur in the commencement of the process of softening.

The process of softening is often regarded as an active one. In the sense of progress towards decay, the term action may not be inappropriate: and in numerous instances in which the process commences from exposure to cold, or other cause of inflammatory action, such a term may fitly imply increased vascular action, and be evidenced in many instances by the occurrence of sudden hæmoptysis and pain over the region affected, and general derangement of the system; but there is certainly a greater mass of cases still in which nothing has occurred to mark the commencement of the process. There are, as is well known, many cases in which extensive destruction of the lung has taken place without the patient having been aware of the existence even of any mischief; but setting aside those which may be regarded as exceptional cases, we do not commonly find anything to mark the first onset of this process in a tubercular mass. Hence, we believe that there are two classes of cases, in one of which there is increased vascular action commonly attended by dyspnœa, pain, hæmoptysis, and a feverish state of the system—the evidences of inflammatory action—whilst in the other the change attracts no attention whatever in its onset, and offers neither general nor local marks of inflammatory action. These two conditions have been commonly regarded as inflammation of a higher or lower order, but it is only with a view to apply our imperfect pathology (such as unquestionably exists in our views of the various kinds of inflammation) that we admit any identity in the two pro-cesses, and nothing is gained beyond mere verbal arrangement by applying the same term to both conditions.

AS TO THE TUBERCLE.

In considering the changes which proceed in tubercle, we must, *in limine*, bear in mind the natural distinction of such a small mass as is inclosed in one cell, and has therefore cell wall and vital struc-tures only upon its circumference, and such a mass of tubercles as is made up of many smaller masses, and which, therefore, has cell walls and inclosed tubercles in many parts of the mass. There are also several other circumstances associated with tubercle in its ten-dency towards health or disease which we must consider; but the two leading ideas involved are the removal of the tubercle from the lungs and the isolation of tubercle in the lungs.

THE REMOVAL OF TUBERCLE FROM THE LUNGS.

It has in all ages been believed that the removal of tuberculous matter by expectoration was the natural course for the cure of this disease. This arose, no doubt, from the analogy of ordinary ab-scesses; for in the time of the early fathers the tuberculous exca-vations were regarded as abscesses, and the natural way to cure an abscess is to evacuate its contents. But although in our day a dis-tinction is drawn between the breaking up of tuberculous masses and ordinary abscesses, it may not be denied that tuberculous mat-ter is removed by expectoration. This process must be confined to two conditions of the disease, viz., the early accumulation of tubercle in each cell, and the period of the formation of a cavity. It is quite conceivable that when tubercle is first deposited, and begins to accumulate, and whilst yet the bronchial tube is open, that portions will escape into the bronchus, but with the exception of a cheesy appearance, we doubt if the material would in that stage be recog-nizable; and we believe that it has never been recognized.[1] There can be no doubt that the epithelial cells constantly undergo destruc-tion and emission, and hence, if tubercle be transformed epithelium, there seems no reason to doubt that this process may still occur, although diminished in activity, by the gradual closing up of the cells and the bronchial tubes, and the diminished vital and physical

---

[1] Dr Radclyffe Hall, in some admirable papers published in the Brit. and For. Med-Chir. Review for 1855 and 1856, speaks of the discovery of degenerated epithelium in the sputa, but he treats of it hypothetically.

actions of the cells. If. therefore, plans be adopted which maintain the patency of the air cells, and increase the vital action of the diseased parts, we see no reason why such accumulation of matter may not be removed in this manner.

At the period of destruction of the lung, and the connection of a cavity with large divisions of the bronchi, it necessarily occurs that as the material disappears and a vacuity is formed, it passes out by expectoration; and as the tissue of the lung becomes destroyed, portions of the yellow elastic fibre are readily found in the expectoration.[1]

The change of the tubercle which leads to this state is known as that of softening of the lung, and occurs nearly always by the admission of the fluid from adjacent portions of the lung, conjoined with changes in the tubercle, and disintegration of the morbid tissue. The softening, as we have elsewhere shown, begins at the centre or the circumference of the mass, according as the tissues in the centre retain pervious bloodvessels; but if it were possible to isolate a single cell filled with tubercle, there could not be a doubt of the softening commencing at the circumference. With the softening, the tubercle undergoes physical changes, by which the cell walls of the tubercle burst, and emit their granular contents, and there are in addition mucous and pus cells. The walls of the several cells, and afterwards those of the lobular membrane, become disintegrated so that the matter contained in the newly-formed cavity, and afterwards in the expectoration, is tubercular, granular, and cellular débris of cell walls, and the tissues of the lung, with mucous and pus cells, often derived from the bronchial mucous membrane, and sometimes with the corpuscles of the blood. As the excavation proceeds, the walls of the cavity become lined with a thick and smooth membrane, secreting a fluid, and called pyogenic membrane, and if the cavity should cease to increase, its walls become thickened by the infiltration of tubercular and other deposits. After a period, the cavity may become empty, and no further tubercular matter be found in it, whilst at the same time it begins to contract in size, if the conditions be favourable and tend to health; but if there be tubercle deposited in the surrounding tissues, the process of excavation commonly continues, and the cavity is less perfectly lined by a membrane, and does not tend to contract, except from the falling in of the walls. This process of contraction is also dependent in part upon the non-existence of pleuritic adhesions to that part of the lung, for it is manifest that so long as the lung at that part is closely held to the walls of the chest, a closure of the cavity is almost impossible.

Hence it appears that expectoration of the tubercle may be presumed to occur throughout the whole period of the disease; for, as

---

[1] It is impossible to entertain too high an opinion of the acuteness and diligence of Prof. Van der Kolk and Dr. Andrew Clark, in their researches upon this subject.

air cells become newly involved in the disease, they may emit tubercle, whilst other cells have become full; and when the destruction of the lung has begun, it is probable that in ordinary cases the expectoration of tubercular matter never ceases until death.

THE ARREST OF TUBERCULIZATION IN THE LUNG.

It has been often remarked that tubercular masses have been found in lungs after death when there was no previous suspicion of their existence, and such prove that the deposition, which had been very restricted, had ceased, and that the tubercular matter (always assuming such masses to be tubercular) had undergone some secondary changes. We do not stay to remark upon the fact of the fewness of such cases in proportion to those in which the disease progresses (so that we must not infer that the condition is common), nor upon the further fact, that as in such cases no careful examination had been made for their detection, we are not entitled to affirm that such conditions could not have been diagnosed, since these questions have been treated of elsewhere, but we take them as simple evidences of the occurrence of one form of cure of tubercle.

OBSOLESCENCE, OR ARREST, OF TUBERCLE.

In this form of arrest of tuberculization we find that a few or many cells have been lost to the lung, and have become filled with, and closed up by, material, whilst the tissues immediately adjoining remain pervious and useful. The tubercle itself has commonly become quite opaque, dry, and calcareous, and the cell walls in which it is inclosed have become dry and detached. In such cases the tubercle, as an irregular nodular mass, may commonly be turned out of the lung, leaving behind it a small irregular cavity.

How far such a condition is due to a diseased action localized to these few cells at the time of the deposition, cannot be determined; but since whatever disorder may affect the whole, may likewise affect a part of the lung, and since such masses are found commonly in the centre of the apex, or at the part of the least mobility of the lung, it is possible that such a localized action may occur. It is, however, more likely, we think, that at the period of deposition of the tubercle in those particular cells, there was a tendency to its deposition in the adjoining cells also, but that the action was thus arrested by the removal of the conditions to which it was owing. It is in this way that we believe the beneficial action of voluntary inspiration proceeds, for whether we consider with M. Piorry that this remedy facilitates the absorption of deposited matter or not, we can have no doubt that its power to maintain the patency and increase the physical and vital action of the cells would tend, at this period, to prevent the extension of the disease, and to give bounds to that then existing. In this state the material may remain without change, or without inducing change, for an indefinite period.

The expectoration of cretaceous tubercle results from such an accumulation of matter, associated with destruction of tissue and the formation of a communication with a tolerably large bronchial tube, and before its expectoration : it becomes again partially softened by the introduction of fluid, so that portions become detached, and are spat up in sizes of from a pin's head to a half a grain of wheat, accompanied usually with an imperfect emulsion of the same material, looking like chalk and water. In such expectoration there will be necessarily the débris of the yellow elastic and other tissues ; but as the process commenced at a distant period, and the tissues have been long shrivelled, their character is far less evident than is observed in recent softening. Yet it may be that recent softening is proceeding in an adjoining part, and the expectorated matter may contain both products.

Tubercle is also subject to other transformations, as, for example, fatty transformation and the production of cholesterine, but these conditions either precede the cretaceous formation, or they are found in such tubercle as tends to softening and destruction of the tissues.

ABSORPTION OF TUBERCLE.

We have just referred to the opinion of so eminent an authority as Piorry, in reference to the promotion of absorption by a particular mode of treatment ; to this we may add the well-ascertained fact of the absorption of inflammatory exudations, although it occurs slowly, and seldom quite perfectly, as presumptive evidence of the absorption of tubercular matter; but it must be recollected that commonly, perhaps, the exudation in inflammation occurs rather between the cell walls than in the cells themselves, that is to say, in the parenchyma of the lung, where it cannot be doubted the more direct vascular actions occur. Yet there is strong evidence in favour of the absorption of tubercular matter from the air cells themselves in the fact that degenerated epithelium in closed cavities must in health be removed by absorption ; and also that under our observation the evidences of the deposition distinctly disappear in a stage so early, that the matter, if removed by expectoration at all, must have passed out, not by a cavity and large bronchus, but by the minute opening of the large bronchial tube.

PART III

TREATMENT.

CHAPTER XXV.

RESTORE THE BULK OF THE BODY BY LESSENING ELIMINATION.

THE SKIN.

In discussing the methods of treatment which are adapted to this disease, we purpose first to consider the indications for treatment, and the best method of fulfilling them, and then to give, in an empirical and categorical manner, a detailed statement of the whole plan which we recommend. It will also be necessary to subdivide the former into those conditions which apply to the system as a whole, including the lungs, and those which refer to the lungs and other organs, &c., as local affections. To these we shall also add chapters upon certain questions which could not be fully treated of under those heads.

We have already shown that we have to do with a disease in which there is commonly diminution of the appetite, flesh, and strength, and increased elimination of fluid and loss of heat; and, that these conditions have arisen almost insensibly, have stealthily increased, and have been long continued. The indications for treatment are, therefore, to restore the bulk of the body, to increase vital action, to regulate muscular and mental labour, and to increase innervation; and to these points we shall give attention in their order.

We have also shown that the term "waste of flesh" comprehends many questions, and particularly those relating to the amount of fluid and fat, as well as the nitrogenous tissues of the body, so that in an attempt to restore the bulk of the body, we must have reference to all these elements. The methods proper for this purpose may be classed under two heads, viz., such as will lessen elimination, and those which increase supply; and of these we will first consider the method whereby elimination may be lessened. The elimination of fluid by the skin can be diminished by numerous methods of treatment.

7

INUNCTION OF OILS AND FATS.

The practice of inunction of the body is very ancient. It was used as a method of healing diseases, as we learn from the Scriptures, and was commonly employed by the Romans and various Eastern nations after the use of the hot bath. It is still employed in both very hot and very cold climates; in the former, when the naked body is exposed to the fierce rays of the sun; and, in the latter, when it is closely enveloped in furs. It is also the practice amongst uncivilized nations to smear the skin with colouring matter and fat; and in reference to the dirty state of the skin in such persons, as well as in those living in cold climates, and with insufficient shelter, it has been remarked that they could not afford to be clean.

In some of these instances, it is possible that the use of the fat may have been simply a matter of luxury; but, generally, we believe it to have had a much deeper meaning, however little it might have been so regarded by those who used it. Thus, inunction after the hot bath would have the effect of lessening the perspiration which followed the bath, and which tended to the injury of those who used the bath excessively, and, therefore, strictly corresponded to the cold wet sheet used in hydropathic establishments, and the cold douche and cold currents of air practised in Turkish baths after the hot bath. When applied to the skin of those whose naked bodies are exposed to the sun, it protects that organ from the chemical rays, by interposing a layer which would be equivalent to an article of clothing; and since the thick and loose clothing which is frequently worn by the Turks and other nations when the external temperature is higher than that of the body, protects the body by preventing the access of the rays of heat, and tends to cool the skin, although it prevents the rapid dispersion of heat from the skin; so, in like manner, will a layer of fat, with or without mineral colouring matter, protect and also cool the skin. The free use of oil and fat externally, and the want of cleanliness of those who live in very cold climates, have also the power to lessen the insensible perspiration, and to offer a non-conductor of heat, which would retard the dispersion of heat, and at the same time prevent the irritating effects of a dry frosty air.

Both of the actions thus described are, we believe, physical. Of the latter action there can be no doubt, since it is demonstrated by the existence of the interposed layers; but, with regard to the former, there are many persons who have not so considered it. It is well known that when a little oil is rubbed over the spiracles, or breathing pores of an insect, the creature dies, because the oil closes the openings and prevents respiration. So it is with the skin, in which the openings of the sweat ducts are closed by the oil or fat, except that, as the air must *enter* the body of the insect by respiration, whilst the perspiration must *pass out* of the body, the former action will be more complete, and the respiration be arrested, whilst the latter action will be only lessened. This action is capable of easy determination, for, if we cover any part of the skin with a thick layer of ointment, we know that neither fluid nor vapour can pass through; but when we reduce the thickness of the layer until it is rendered imperfect, we find that fluid will at length be emitted. Hence, we believe, that there can be no doubt of the fact, that in both cases alike, the principal action of the oil or fat is physical.

Then, again, there are many who believe that the fat becomes absorbed by the skin, and plays a part in the general and local[1] nutrition of the body; and in proof, reference is made to the disappearance of the oil or ointment after friction. We admit the latter as a fact, but do not equally admit the former as an inference. Fat or oil disappears, in great part at least, because it is rubbed off by the clothing, or runs off by the liquefying effect of the heat of the body, and, of necessity, a certain portion will enter every opening in the skin, and thus temporarily disappear; but it will be observed that there is no anatomical arrangement of the skin whereby the oil can be carried into the general circulation; neither is there the presence of the alkali, which, in the bile and pancreatic juice, is understood to be essential to form an emulsion of fat. The only openings upon the skin are those of the sebaceous glands and sweat ducts, whilst all the surface is covered by a material which is nonvascular, and the perspiration is either neutral or slightly acid. Hence, there are grave doubts as to the true absorption of fat by the skin, and of conversion into nutritive material, to be employed either locally or through the general system.[2]

In the disease now under consideration, the inunction of oil is useful when there is excessive elimination of fluid by the skin, by restraining that action, and also by offering, in some degree, a protection against external agents acting upon a highly sensitive structure. These actions are mechanical, and will, therefore, be more or less efficient as the fat more or less completely covers the pores of the skin. Hence, in the employment of inunction it is requisite to find a material which will not readily be removed from the skin, and to use it in such a manner that a layer of fat shall always cover the skin. In reference to the material, we may cite the employment of olive oil, cod-liver oil, neat's-foot oil, and lard.

Olive oil has the great advantage of not offering an offensive

---

[1] Dr. F. W. Mackenzie stated at the Medical Society of London that he had known deposition of fat about the chest to follow the local external use of cod-liver oil; but if morbific putrid matters applied to the skin do not gain entrance into the circulation unless there be abrasion of the skin, it is not easy to see how fats would find admission; and if they should be admitted, it yet remains to be proved in what manner they are deposited locally in the place near to which they were externally applied.

[2] This is practically admitted by the absence of all attempts to nourish the system through the skin in cases in which deglutition is almost impossible. If the skin can absorb fats, there is a presumption that it could absorb other aliments, as milk and wine—practically a *reductio ad absurdum*.

odour, and of being a substance of ordinary use to some part of the body, and one therefore with which the public is familiarly acquainted ; but it has the disadvantage of rarefying by the heat of the body to so great an extent, that it runs off the skin, and is most readily wiped away. Hence it is impossible to keep the skin covered with a layer of it, unless some plan be adopted whereby it may be almost constantly reapplied. *Cod-liver oil* and *neat's-foot oil* possess the great advantage of viscidity, and remain upon the warm skin for a much longer period than olive oil. Hence they are much more fitted for the object which we have in view, but the odour which arises from them prevents their general use.

Lard, being solid fat, is better adapted for the purposes of inunction than liquid oils, and possessing but little odour, it is but slightly offensive. The addition of a portion of mutton suet renders it less liable to be removed by the heat of the body, and the ordinary spermaceti ointment is an excellent remedy. Hence, of the substances named, olive oil and lard are those to which the least objection is advanced by patients, whilst the former is the least, and the latter the most fitted for the purpose in a physical point of view.

In the method of inunction it is important to attend to the following rules : 1st. That the ointment shall be rubbed over every part of the body not less than twice a day, and so rubbed that the aim shall be, not to induce the largest amount of absorption, but to cover the skin in the most perfect manner, and to leave a layer of fat upon it. 2d. When thus covered, the layer would remain for many hours if the skin could be left uncovered and free from contact with external objects, but as this cannot be, at least in our climate, a considerable portion of it will be removed whenever any clothing is put on. Hence it is necessary that there be a dress worn which shall cover nearly the whole skin in one piece, and worn so long a time without change, that the inner surface becoming oily may the less tend to absorb the fat from the skin. Perhaps the best material for this purpose is a tolerably thick twilled calico, without a nap, and it may be worn either as a long chemise, or be made to fit the body as vest and drawers. 3d. The plan should be pursued for a number of days, say seven or ten, without any intermission, or for as long a time as the patient will tolerate it, if the skin still require it. It is desirable to allow a few days to elapse after the treatment has been discontinued, lest the patient should become weary of it, and then the inunction may be renewed and repeated in like manner for a long period, if it should be necessary. 4th. Care must be taken not to allow the body to remain long uncovered during the inunction, unless it be summer weather, lest cold be taken ; but if the application be rapidly performed, time will not be allowed in which injury may occur, and the ointment itself will tend to prevent cold.

It has been affirmed that persons who handle oil and fat daily are less frequently afflicted with phthisis than other persons, and whilst such general statements can never be admitted as grounds for theory, it is probable that the constant oiling of the exposed parts of the body—as the hands, arms, face, and neck by cloth-workers, butchers, and others, may prevent the skin of these parts being too active. In the cases of butchers, it is well known that the ordinary tendency is to an inactive state of the skin, as shown by the colour, heat, and moderate dryness of that organ, whatever may be the causes to which that may be due.

THE APPLICATION OF COLD WATER.

It would appear at first sight that the application of cold to a skin in which perspiration is proceeding, and which possesses great sensitiveness to cold would be injurious; but we have been taught of late years that, within certain limits, these changes may be effected with rapidity and impunity. The object to be had in view, however, is not to lower the temperature of the skin, although that may be a necessary condition to the attainment of our object, but to remove the atonic or relaxed state of the skin, with which an unusual tendency to perspiration is always associated, and to restore the skin to its normal tone. For this purpose cold is very efficacious, from its known property of contracting vital tissues, and the chief care must be to apply it in such a manner that tone may be given without materially lowering the temperature of the skin. In exercising this care, it is better to use water of the temperature of the room, viz., from 50° to 60°, according to the season of the year, and either to plunge the whole body at once into it, or to apply a small quantity of it as quickly as possible to the whole surface. If the plunge bath be used, it should be expeditiously effected, and friction be applied directly afterwards, and this may be .performed either in open water or at baths. When sponging is preferred, it should be effected night and morning, and care be taken that the sponge or towel does not retain so much water that when pressed upon the body, the water shall trickle in streams over the skin. We prefer a towel for this purpose, and after it has been dipped into the water and pressed, so as to leave but little water in it, it should be quickly applied and reapplied to all parts of the body. The whole operation need not occupy more than one minute and a half, and as the towel becomes less cold after it has first touched the body, the shock is not considerable. In order to produce the effect which we desire, it must be dipped several times into the water. It is customary with many persons to bathe the chest, or some small part of the body which is ordinarily covered with clothing, and to leave the greater part of the body unbathed. We think this both a useless and a dangerous practice in the conditions now under consideration, for the object can be attained only when the whole skin is influenced, and there is much greater liability to take cold when the temperature of one part of the skin is lowered, and that of the other parts remains high.

There is still some unfounded prejudice against the free use of cold water, on the ground of a supposed liability to take cold under its use. We grant that if only a part of the skin be so acted upon, and the naked body be exposed to a cool temperature for some time, this is very liable to occur; but when the whole body is acted upon at the same time—as by the shower or plunge bath, or by the wet sheet—there is not the least danger, and in proportion as the temperature of the skin has been rapidly lowered, so will the glow of heat be felt when the skin has been dried and covered.

On the same ground there are many who use lukewarm water, and others, who by the routine of the hydropathic treatment, precede the use of cold by the employment of the hot bath, but in the conditions in question both plans are injurious. The use of the warm water would not afford the contractile action which we desire, and by the evaporation which would be set up, would be likely to give cold to a sensitive skin, whilst the hot-bath cannot be useful in any case in which the skin is ordinarily too active, and where the sole design is to lessen the activity.

There is a common belief that the use of salt water is attended with less liability to cold than that of simple water, and, although this is based upon opinion only, we attach value to it. It is also probable that the salt itself possesses a stimulating property, and is, therefore, well fitted to diminish the atonicity of the skin. In our ordinary treatment we advise the use of a small quantity of a cold saturated solution of either common or rock salt, with a towel, as above directed, or the use of the cold plunge bath, either of simple or salt water. The former may be practised at every season of the year, and the good effects which the patients attribute to it are universal.

In the cases in which we employ inunction, we also recommend the use of the salt and water sponging in the intervals during which the inunction is omitted.

CLOTHING.

In the conditions of the skin now under consideration, we have to guard against unduly lessening or increasing the temperature by clothing, and of increasing perspiration. The rule to be observed is to use so much clothing as will allow the skin to be moderately cool, without the patient having the sensation of cold; but in the cases in which the extremities are cold, it is essential that the clothing of these parts be abundant.

The period when excess of clothing is ordinarily injurious is the night time, when it is often the habit to protect the sensitive skin by much clothing, and as the tendency to perspire is always the greatest when the vital actions are the lowest, viz., from 3 to 5 A.M., it will necessarily occur that perspiration will follow, and the skin in the early morning will be in its most relaxed and sensitive condition.

Others have acquired the habit of unduly covering the body during the day, whenever there is the least exposure to cool air, either by wearing two flannel shirts, or two waistcoats, or an overcoat, or by several layers of flannel or skins on various parts of the chest. Such persons are afraid to undress on account of the shock which they experience when the cool air comes in contact with their soft and sensitive skin, and it not unfrequently happens, in the cases in question, that when they are divested of their clothing there is a cloud of vapour surrounding the body.

Hence in both of these conditions there is excess of clothing, and it is requisite that the bathing with salt and water be employed, at the same time that the quantity of clothing is lessened, so that the sensitiveness of the skin be reduced as the exposure to the cooler air is enforced. It is also advisable that the patient do not sleep on a feather bed, and that the bed clothing be gradually lessened.

The use of flannel shirts is much more general than it was in former years, but it is yet very common to find persons in the early stage of phthisis who have never worn them. In an inquiry upon 1000 patients we found that $14\frac{1}{2}$ per cent., had never worn flannel upon the skin, and that a further $10\frac{1}{2}$ per cent. had worn for periods not longer than six months. Hence it may be affirmed, that 25 per cent. of the cases of both sexes had not worn flannel upon the skin in health; but if the women alone are considered, the proportion was no less than 39 per cent.

We attach the greatest importance to the use of flannel shirts, chiefly on the ground that woollen being a bad conductor of heat, they prevent the immediate accession of cold air to the chest under conditions of sudden exposure. We regard them, therefore, as preventives of disease, and in that light it is manifest that a closely woven fabric is the most fitted for the purpose, and that no amount of loose and more open external clothing can offer the same protection as an ill-conducting fabric which closely fits the body and is applied immediately to the skin. The thickness and weight of the material is of far less consequence than its close manufacture, its good nap, and its tight covering to the whole chest; and hence, while the wove shirts of the present day have the advantage of more closely fitting the body, the fine Welsh flannel is a more efficient material.

A woollen shirt, of whatever kind, which is worn threadbare, or which does not closely fit the body, is of little value.

In connection with this part of the subject is that of defective clothing. It rarely happens that defective clothing is associated with an active skin, except when conjoined with living in close, and therefore heated, rooms, and with great exhaustion of system from whatever cause. Hence in such cases the problem is a complicated one, but if the skin be cool and the extremities cold, with deficient clothing, it is manifest that the clothing should be increased, and the risk of inducing a more active condition of the skin be averted by the use of the salt and water bath.

It may be of advantage to introduce here a few remarks on the use of clothing which is impenetrable to moisture. We think we are right in affirming that, whilst the use of Indian-rubber goloshes has increased, and that of waterproof coats has perhaps not diminished materially, the periods during which they are worn are now more restricted than formerly. It is manifest that by so much as they are fitted to defend the body from external wet, by so much do they necessarily prevent the egress of the vapour from the body, so that it is common to find that the smooth Indian-rubber surface of the inside of a coat, which has been worn when buttoned closely and during exertion, is covered with moisture, whilst the under clothing is more or less saturated, the temperature of the surface materially increased, and the skin rendered soft and very active. So, also, in reference to the feet, when goloshes or patent-leather boots are worn, as the wet state of the socks, and the soft, shrivelled, and sometimes abraded state of the skin of the feet will prove. The first effect of the use of these articles of clothing is, therefore, to increase the action of the skin, and, by retaining the heat, to increase the temperature of the surface; but the effect at a later period is to give a sensation of cold and to increase the sensibility of the skin. All persons who wear goloshes for lengthened periods find the feet cold.

Hence, in the conditions of disease to which we now refer, it is injurious to wear waterproof materials of clothing, except under urgent circumstances, and then their use should be discontinued as early as possible. When in use they should not thoroughly envelop any part. Under the ordinary conditions of life we regard them as injurious.

EXPOSURE TO THE ATMOSPHERE.

Regulated, but yet free, exposure to the ordinary variations of the atmosphere is to be commended.

Moderately free exposure to a cool atmosphere at all periods of the day acts upon the skin in a manner almost identical with that described under the head of cold bathing. It will be in vain to attempt to increase the tone of the skin by the infrequent use of cold water, unless at the same time the patient be induced to quit his room, where the air is stagnant and the temperature high, and to seek the open air with its vigorous breezes and lower temperature. We are of opinion that nothing tends so much to induce the unfavourable condition of skin now under consideration, as the state of the atmosphere in close rooms and in crowded houses, and that all such persons ought to spend a very large portion of the day in the open air and in moderately exposed positions.

It is highly probable that in former years the disease in question offered more frequent evidences of an inflammatory type than is now observed, and consequently demanded a sheltered house and a residence in a warmer climate; but, however true this may have been, we affirm that in the ordinary cases of the disease there is now nothing whatever to forbid the free exposure of the body to the external air. There are many who depreciate exposure to all weathers, and seek shelter whenever there is a little rain or the wind blows somewhat cold. We, however, do not see any ground for this, and if suitable clothing be used and exertion made, we would place little restriction as to the kind of weather. There can be no doubt that warm and moist weather is the least to be desired in the conditions now under consideration, and as little that a dry and cool, and even frosty, air is the most advantageous.

The universal objection which exists to the east wind must be based upon truth, however difficult it may be to assign a proper reason for it. There can be no doubt as to that wind being a pre-eminently dry and drying one, as the dry and harsh skin, and the dry tongue and throat of many persons during its occurrence testify. So far an easterly wind will clearly be less injurious to the conditions of skin now under consideration, than in the ordinary state of that organ, but otherwise it may be injurious.

FOOD.

The observations which have been commonly made in reference to the action of food upon the skin, are such as have followed its use when it disagreed with the system, and hence have been attributed to a diseased and not to a healthy action. These observations were no doubt correct, and were due to the cause indicated, but they also show the direction of the action of foods under normal conditions, for it must follow, that both in health and disease alike, the direction of the action of food would be the same, whilst the degree of the action might be so different that in one case it would be compatible with health, and in the other would so exceed the bounds of health as to cause disease.

Thus it has been observed that alcohols dry the skin, and particularly the stronger forms of them, as brandy and rum, and, in our experiments, it was recorded by one of the gentlemen under its influence, that the effect was as drying as an east wind.[1] This occurs both with the ordinary and unusual doses of the alcohol, but more readily on some occasions than on others. It is also fully admitted, that in fevers, when the skin is dry and parched, and in certain forms of derangement of the liver, when the skin is commonly dry,

[1] Phil. Trans. 1859.

alcohols cannot be tolerated, whilst in conditions such as those under consideration they are well borne, and are useful.

Fats, also, when they do not agree, but cause indigestion, are followed by headache and dry skin, as was known to Hippocrates, whatever may be the kind of fat, and whether it be taken separately or in the combination found in milk or in artificial cooking. This was noticed by us in our experiments, and also that the tendency of flesh meat in general was to lessen the action of the skin. Coffee was invariably seen to dry the skin in our experiments.

Hence, in the conditions now under discussion, some of the forms of alcohol, coffee, fats, and milk, are especially fitted for employment, and it is a familiar and analogous fact, that they tend to induce constipation. The old and well-approved combination of rum and milk, or brandy and milk, in the dose of two teaspoonfuls, or a dessertspoonful, of spirit to half-a-pint of milk is very proper, and particularly in the early morning, when the skin is commonly very active. During the day no form is better than that of home-brewed ale, when not too strong; or, failing this, good Dublin stout; but the dose should never be so great as to affect the head, nor the use of it continued after the due effect upon the skin has been produced.

In reference to the night hours, when perspirations more usually occur, we have found that food of almost any kind will tend to lessen the elimination, but the most suitable kinds are coffee and milk, together or separately, and not unfrequently cold tea has been equally beneficial. All these substances have the common effect of increasing the action of the heart temporarily, and at the period in question, the pulsation and all the vital actions are extremely reduced. Whether the effect upon the skin is produced in this manner we do not stay to inquire.

On the other hand, it is a matter of common observation that some other kinds of food do not lessen but increase the action of the skin. This is the case with warm water, tea, bread, and fresh vegetables, and whilst the two latter must be eaten, the second should be usually avoided.

MEDICINES.

The action of medicines has been ascertained for the most part by the empirical method just referred to when discussing the influence of food, and it is well established that certain substances promote, and others lessen the action of the skin. This has been proved both by their ill effects when they have not agreed, and by their unfitness in certain states of the system. Thus it has been shown that iron and its salts, with zinc and many other mineral preparations known as tonics, with acids and vegetable tonics in general, lessen the action of the skin, and are particularly fitted for cases in which the skin is active, and cannot be administered in febrile and other conditions in which the skin is dry. Hence recently our friend Dr. Robert Dickson has introduced the oxide of zinc as a remedy for night perspirations. The action of iodine upon the functions of the skin has not been well determined, but it is highly probable it lessens the activity of that organ, as is found in the cases of general struma, in which it is very beneficial.

Hence in the conditions under consideration all these remedies are applicable, and the ordinary composition of a preparation of iron, with acid, and a vegetable bitter, is manifestly the best with which we are at present acquainted. There is much difference in practice as to the precise form of a metal which shall be given, and much ingenuity has been exhibited of late years to provide salts of iron to meet these views, and also the supposed requirements of practice. We cannot but think that the differences of action are in a degree rather matters of opinion than of fact, and in practice one or two forms seem to fulfil almost every indication. Such, for example, as the sesquichloride of iron, and the citrate of iron with quinine; but, of the two, we ordinarily prefer the former in doses of 15 to 25 minims thrice a day.

Lead is also a powerful agent for the purpose now under consideration, as may be inferred from its power to arrest sanguineous and alvine discharges, although it has not hitherto been employed with the express object here indicated. It is an old remedy in the treatment of phthisis, but within the last few years only have its merits been brought clearly before the profession. M. Beau, the present distinguished physician to *La Charité*, following the observations of Hildebrand, has very recently recommended its employment in all stages of the malady.[1] His data are purely empirical, for the idea was derived from the alleged fact that persons engaged in the operations of lead mines and white lead works are not very liable to phthisis, and as such persons are liable to the affection known as lead colic, M. Beau believes it to be essential to produce a similar condition in every phthisical patient. This condition implies lessened elimination, and constipation, with great diminution of the power of the cerebro-spinal system of nerves, for such a condition is indicated in the distended state of the bowels in painter's colic, and demonstrated in the hanging wrists and other evidences of paralysis which occur in more advanced cases of the lead poisoning.

We must be exceedingly cautious how we admit such statements as grounds for treatment in any, but particularly in so important a class of cases as phthisis, since the very basis of the infrequency of phthisis in the class referred to is not by any means established, and since all empirical observations are liable to error, both in their interpretation and in the extension of the class of persons in which they are observed. The most that could be fairly inferred from the facts already known is, that in some persons the influence of lead may be beneficial as a prophylactic of phthisis, and it would remain to define the characters of that class. Our own belief of the action of the lead, and of the class of persons in which it would be useful, has already been expressed, and hence we regard it in no wise as a specific remedy in phthisis, but as one which may be advantageously employed in a selected class of cases in the early stage with a view to remove certain collateral conditions.

We do not recommend the adoption of M. Beau's plan of treatment, neither do we think that any physician to a public charity in England would feel himself justified in inducing consequences so serious as those pointed out by M. Beau, or in so expending the precious time afforded for the treatment of the case within the walls of an hospital. M. Beau considers, as we have above stated, that in order to obtain the good effects of the lead, it is necessary to continue it until constipation and lead colic are obtained. Within that degree he states that the action is rather unfavourable, since it lessens the appetite, is liable to disorder the digestion, and, when given by the stomach, produces diarrhœa. Moreover, he adds gastralgia, gastric cough, and dyspnœa to this list of preliminary evils. But after the constitutional influences of the lead have been attained, M. Beau asserts that there is improvement in the cough and all the general symptoms, and the change in the lung disease may amount almost to a cure. He states, also, that of twelve persons so treated, the disease was checked and the physical signs improved in four, the disease had almost disappeared in four, and two others were apparently altogether cured. He prescribes the carbonate of lead in 2 grain doses, daily adding 2 grains on each succeeding day until 12 grains daily are given, or the lead poisoning is effected.

We believe the remedy to be useful in the class of cases where there is emaciation, due chiefly to a constitutional disposition to excessive elimination, and where, as a consequence, there is a diminution in the heat of the body and the vital powers ; but it should be given rather in an intermitting than a continuous manner.

There is, however, a temporary condition of the perspiration, which in our judgment modifies the kind of treatment here advised, and which it may be proper to refer to here, viz : the acid odour of the perspiration which is observed in many cases. This condition is oftentimes very marked, and on inquiry it will be found that it has attracted the attention of the patient. It is also more common in the night than in the day perspiration. It suffices to divide the class of cases now under consideration into two classes, so far as the treatment is concerned ; for we have noticed that those on whom perspirations, whether by night or day, are profuse, acids and mineral tonics do not diminish the action of the skin, whilst in such cases the use of the ordinary saline medicine containing acetate of ammonia, or of a combination of salts of soda and potash, soon remove the sour odour and the perspirations together. There is some variation in the cases, so that in one class the ammonia salt is more efficacious than the soda and potash ; and such for the most part are those who experience chilliness and severe sense of alternations of temperature, as in a common cold, whilst in a few cases the plan now indicated is of no avail. Our ordinary plan is to administer the alkalies or neutral salts in cases where the perspiration possesses the sour odour, and when there is much debility, we have commonly found that the ammonio-chloride of iron is the best of all the tonic preparations. This condition is temporary, and after a period the treatment required is that which is fitted for those in whom there is no acid odour; but we have known many cases in which the continued use of a saline for several weeks was attended by much comfort and increase of strength. As an instance of marked improvement from the plan of treatment here recommended, we cite the following case of early phthisis.

There was constant and excessive elimination of acid by the skin, without other symptoms than excessive and general exhaustion and wasting, and it did not progress satisfactorily during three or four months. Under the influence of the combination of potass and soda, he had a very profuse sweating, accompanied by an exceedingly acid and acrid odour; and obtained immediate and almost marvellous relief.

J. E., a young, single man, aged 20, engaged in a grocer's shop in the country, had complained for three months of bad appetite, with brown tongue, foul breath, and slight emaciation. There was slight hæmoptysis occasionally, with slight dyspnœa. There was scarcely any cough, but the throat had been sore from the commencement of his disease. The general expression of the symptoms was nervous exhaustion and muscular debility. The chest presented the slightest shade of dulness on percussion, and lessened respiration on the left side.

On August 21st, he began to take iron, with a mineral acid and quinia. Cod-liver oil was added on August 28th. In September he continued in the same state, but with a little increase of cough and debility. In October, the cough continued but he felt a little general improvement. There was also a little pain in the left breast. His state was becoming more anæmic; and the iron, being intermitted for a time, was renewed in November. During all this period he took out-of-door exercise, used salt-and-water ablutions, and was directed to take milk and other nutritive kinds of food at short intervals during the day and night.

Thus three months passed away without any visible improvement, and the progress of the lung-disease appeared imminent. At the end of November, however, he had a most profuse sweating during four nights, in frosty weather, accompanied by an exceedingly sour and acrid odour, which appeared to be the crisis of his condition; for, under the influence of bicarbonate of potass and gentian, he improved most rapidly, and the increase of perspiration, with its acid state, ceased in December. Throughout January he continued to improve, and became again cheerful, active, and strong; and the cod-liver oil being again prescribed at the beginning of February (it having disagreed with him in the early part of his attack), caused so much improvement in a fortnight, that he was led to look upon it as the principal means of his restoration to health. It is very probable that, had the alkaline treatment been begun earlier, we should have been spared some anxiety.

Cases are also met with in which the perspiration is profuse and of a very sour odour, and does not yield to treatment, and in such the disease commonly progresses rapidly. When the perspiration is not acid, the ordinary forms of mineral and vegetable tonics, with acids, are well fitted to lessen the action of the skin.

CHAPTER XXVI.

RESTORE THE BULK OF THE BODY BY LESSENING ELIMINATION.

THE KIDNEYS AND BOWELS.

THERE is undoubtedly a close relation between the action of the skin and the kidneys, so that any increase or decrease in the elimination by the skin will be attended by the converse condition in the kidneys. Hence, in the condition of disease now under consideration, in which there is commonly increased action of the skin, the quantity of urine evolved is seldom in any marked excess.

There are, however, periods when the kidneys eliminate large quantities of urine, either from a sudden change in the relations of the skin to the kidneys, or from some other cause acting directly through the latter organs. There are also numerous instances in which the amount of urine is unduly increased by drinking large quantities of water or weak tea, and since the ordinary effect of drinking fluids alone is to cause an elimination of more fluid than they have afforded to the body, the result is to produce excessive elimination. Moreover, many persons indulge in the use of gin or other alcohols, which tend directly to increase elimination by the kidneys.

In the treatment of the early stage of phthisis, it is very desirable that the fluids taken should be duly restricted, that they should not be of a nature to increase elimination, and that they should be administered with solid food, which may require them for its solution, and will temporarily fix them in the tissues. It is highly probable that the evil effect of gin-drinking is evident in this manner before the further condition of diseased kidneys is induced, and is thereby one of the causes of phthisis. It must also be admitted that the indiscriminate use of large quantities of Spa waters before breakfast tends largely to injury in this direction in persons suffering from the condition now under discussion, since at that period of the day, and when taken without food, simple water is a most powerful diuretic.[1]

The patients frequently express a desire for much fluid to satisfy thirst, and so far it is indicative of excessive elimination, for both perspiration and diuresis, when in large excess, induce thirst. In such cases the plan of treatment is to lessen the elimination of fluid, and then the thirst will disappear.

When the excessive elimination of fluid by the kidneys is associated with disease of the kidney, its prevention is seldom within our reach ; and as it is rarely found in the early stage of phthisis, and has no necessary relation to that disease, we do not purpose to enter upon its discussion.

There is much variation in the habits of men as to the frequency with which dejections from the bowels naturally occur, and consequently as to the quantity of alvine excretion. There is also very great tolerance of these variations, so that we have known many persons in good health who have been accustomed to only one dejection in ten or fourteen days, whilst others have alvine evacuations twice or thrice a day. It is, therefore, impossible to lay down any rule which may be considered as necessary to health, or to affirm that the ordinary daily evacuation is much more natural than a less frequent one. It is no doubt, in fact, dependent upon the amount and kind of food eaten, and the amount of food which has been transformed ; for the larger the amount of refuse and unused food in the bowel, the more necessary it is to have a frequent dejection. But in the disease in question, where the appetite is somewhat diminished, there is perhaps less than the ordinary necessity for a daily evacuation. When the food is habitually long retained, it may be inferred that its nutritive qualities are more perfectly extracted than would have occurred in the same person with a daily evacuation ; whilst frequent evacuations always contain a large amount of nutritive material. Hence, in ordinary cases, we would not advise a rigid conformity with the ordinary rule of a daily evacuation. In this matter the ordinary habits of the patient must be duly considered, and it not unfrequently happens that frequent dejections have been the rule, or that this condition has existed for some time ; but even then, unless other circumstances contra-indicate it, we would rather lessen the frequency of the act ; and where there are frequent dejections, to which may be in part attributed the condition under discussion, the first object should be to arrest it.

We do not here refer to the conditions of the bowel which commonly give rise to diarrhœa, since they belong to a later period of the disease than we purpose to embrace.

[1] Phil. Trans., 1861.

CHAPTER XXVII.

RESTORE THE BULK OF THE BODY BY INCREASING THE SUPPLY.

DEFICIENCY OF NITROGEN IN ADOLESCENCE.

HAVING now shown the degree of activity in the eliminating actions of the body, and the methods whereby it may be restrained, and thus arrest the loss of weight and bulk of the body, which is a common feature in this disease, we now proceed to show how far the emaciation may be lessened by a positive increase in the amount of food supplied.

It will be well understood, *in limine,* that it is one thing to place food in the stomach, and another to have it duly digested and transformed, so that only a little may pass off by the bowel; but there is, nevertheless, a close relationship between the appetite for food and the power of the system to transform the food, and, as a practical rule, if the patient can be induced to increase the quantity of food taken, we may be sure that there will be an increase in the quantity transformed, although not necessarily in exact proportion to the increase of the food. The former question we shall hereafter consider more at large when speaking of the increase in the vital actions, and shall here refer only to the latter, or the increase of the quantity of food.

We have already stated that there is commonly some diminution in the amount of food eaten, and in addition to this, we may affirm that, whatever may be the relation of the present to the usual quantity of food, there is in the cases in question very commonly an absolute defect in the required quantity. It is impossible to lay down any general rule which shall be applicable to individual cases, and therefore, to some extent, each case must be determined by itself, and a comparison made between the present and the usual quantity of food; but yet there are certain general grounds which are widely applicable.

We have elsewhere shown that the nitrogenous element in food[1] is necessary both for the supply of material to be fixed in the nitrogenous tissues, and for the true transformation of the hydro-carbons; and there is the most serious reason to believe that this element is commonly deficient in the food of the persons to whose condition we are now referring.

At the period of life when youth is passing into adolescence, and when so large a portion of mankind fall into phthisis, there is such a change in the dietary that the amount of nitrogen supplied is greatly lessened in proportion to the weight of the body, and the

[1] Phil. Trans., 1859.

greatest liability to a diminution below that required by the system at this period of growth. Thus taking the amount of urea evolved to represent the amount of nitrogen ingested, we have shown, in our work on the cyclical changes of the human system, that there are 5, 6, or 7 grains of urea to each pound weight of body, at three, four, or five years of age; but it is reduced to 2, 3, or 4 grains at sixteen or eighteen years of age. This is chiefly to be attributed to the diminution in the supply of milk without a corresponding increase in the supply of other nitrogenous foods, and at the same time there is an increase of the hydro-carbon starch, which, as above mentioned, demands the addition of nitrogen for its due assimilation. The proportion of nitrogen to the carbon in bread is 1 to 22, but in milk it is 1 to 11; so that for every pound of milk omitted, there should be two pounds of bread added. The addition of meat which is made when the supply of milk is lessened is generally quite inadequate to meet the loss thus occasioned; for if a fair proportion of fat and lean meat be taken, the quantity of nitrogen per ounce scarcely exceeds 8 grains, whilst that in good bread is nearly as much, and it would require 5½ oz. of good uncooked fat and lean meat to supply as much nitrogen as is found in one pint of good new milk.

We know that at the period in question, when the quantity of milk is reduced one or two pints daily, there is not commonly an equivalent increase in meat and bread, and hence this most essential vital excitant falls into defect. This we believe to be the case in all classes of society, and to constitute one of the most common causes of this disease. In the rich it is customary for tea and coffee, which offer scarcely any nitrogen, with but a small portion of milk, to constitute the breakfast of the young man or woman, who a few years earlier ate one pint of milk at that meal, containing 44 grs. nitrogen, and a quantity of bread scarcely less than that eaten in adolescence, whilst the children of the poor are frequently compelled to live throughout the day upon little but tea and bread.

As a general rule, it may be laid down that the quantity of nitrogen supplied for each pound weight of body, from fourteen to twenty years of age, should not be less than 1½ gr., and that of carbon 25 grs.; so that, if we consider the weight of the body to vary from 90 lbs. to 150 lbs. in that period, the total daily quantity would be 135 grs. to 275 grs. of nitrogen, and 5 oz. to 8½ oz. of carbon.

The dietary which should be supplied may be thus stated. Three pints of milk; 1¼ lb. of bread; 6 oz. of uncooked meat (equal to 4 oz. of cooked meat); ¾ lb. of potatoes; 1½ oz. of butter and 3 oz. of uncooked bacon, or 4 oz. of eggs. This would give the following quantity of nitrogen:—

	Nitrogen.
3 pints of milk, new and good, grains .	132
6 ozs. meat (fat and lean)	48
20 ozs. of bread	135
12 ozs. potatoes	9

344

Hence we would supply upwards of 300 grs. of nitrogen per day, and thus be in excess of the daily requirements of the system, and allow a considerable quantity to be fixed in the tissues of the body as they increase in bulk. In order that this large quantity of food may be taken and duly digested, it is requisite that it be wisely distributed over the twenty-four hours, and to this we attach the greatest importance.

But there are very many cases in which the patient is unable to take sufficient food to supply so large a quantity of nitrogen, and it is of great consequence to meet this deficiency. This is largely effected by Bouchardat's various preparations of glutenized foods recently introduced into this country by G. Van Abbott & Co., which we have extensively used in our experimental researches and in the dietary of phthisical patients. These preparations are— gluten bread, which is prepared in slices, and must be toasted and eaten hot; semola, the ground gluten bread containing 80 per cent. of gluten, and chocolate, the best quality of which contains 10 per cent. of gluten.

In our experiments we found that $1\frac{1}{2}$ oz. of gluten bread, when taken alone, increased the emission of carbonic acid to the maximum extent of 1.04 and 1.07 gr. per minute, and maintained the effect for fully three hours. Two ounces of gluten bread, taken in the morning, caused an increase of 62 grs. of urea during the day; $1\frac{1}{2}$ oz. of the best gluten chocolate caused an increase in the quantity of carbonic acid evolved of 2 grs. per minute, with the increase enduring for about 3 hours.

As gluten contains about 16 per cent. of nitrogen, it is evident that if the gluten bread and the semola contain 80 per cent. of gluten, there will be as much nitrogen supplied in 1 oz. as is contained in $1\frac{1}{4}$ pint of milk or 7 oz. of ordinary bread, and that we have in them most valuable agents. The gluten bread may be eaten like ordinary toast with any meal, whilst the semola may be prepared with milk, and taken separately or in puddings. In the treatment of consumptive patients we attach very great value to the use of these substances. Their action is to increase the activity of all vital functions, since, by so largely increasing the evolution of carbonic acid, they must aid in the transformation of starchy and other hydro-carbonaceous foods, and at the same time the nitrogen supplies the elements requisite for the formation of the tissues of the body. Hence they increase assimilation.

In cases of consumption and general debility, it is our practice to recommend the daily use of 4 oz. of gluten bread or semola and two quantities of gluten chocolate, in addition to, or to supply a deficiency in, the quantity of nitrogenous food just referred to; and we are able to affirm that the results have been highly satisfactory.

SCHEME OF DAILY DIET.

We have already shown that the vital actions are greatly reduced during the night, and that in phthisis the night depression far exceeds that observed in health. Hence it is of prime importance to supply food in the night as well as in the day, and the following is the scheme which we ordinarily recommend :—

1. Immediately on awaking in the early morning, ½ a pint of milk (hot if possible), alone, or with chocolate added, with bread and butter.
2. For breakfast : ¾ pint of milk with coffee, chocolate, or oatmeal, and eggs or bacon in addition.
3. At 11 A. M. ½ a pint of milk, or of good beef tea, made from ox heads or shins, with bread and butter.
4. An early dinner, with plenty of meat, and milk and egg pudding.
5. An early tea, consisting of milk with coffee or chocolate, and bread and butter.
6. An early supper of ¾ pint of milk, with oatmeal or chocolate, and bread and butter; or two eggs with bread and butter, and milk to drink.
7. During the night a cup of milk and a little bread and butter to be placed by the bedside and to be eaten if the patient should awake.

By this mode a much larger quantity of food may be taken than would be possible if the food were given only at the usual meal hours, and as it will be taken in small quantities, the system will not be oppressed by it, and the vital actions will not be allowed to subside. It is a dietary which allows a considerable quantity of nutritious material, both nitrogenous and hydro-carbonaceous, to be stored up in the system, since it is rich in both classes of nutriment.

SPECIAL ARTICLES OF FOOD.

We think it of great importance that there should be a considerable amount of fat taken, whatever may be the quantity of starch supplied, since it is manifest from common experience that starch alone cannot meet the requirements of the system in reference to this class of food. The dietary just recommended supplies nearly 3 oz. of butter in the milk, and this added to the butter eaten with the bread, would amount to 5 oz. daily. The meat, when well fed, offers upon the whole beast from 25 to 50 per cent. of fat, so that with 6 oz. of fresh meat we shall supply about 2 oz. of fat, giving a total daily supply of fat of 7 oz.

The essential consideration in the dietary for patients in early phthisis is abundance of nitrogenous and fatty foods, with such an addition of starchy foods as may be necessary for admixture with the fat, and this we would in the most serious manner urge upon the attention of all having charge of such cases.   There are doubtless many other articles of food which enter into ordinary dietaries, and which might be properly introduced into this one, besides these now indicated; and amongst these we may mention gelatin, isinglass, Irish moss, and various modern preparations of grain, as corn-flour and semolina.

There is a prevalent belief amongst scientific men that gelatin does not aid in the work of nutrition.   This has been derived from the results of the inquiries of the " Gelatin Commission" in France, which showed that animals could not live on bones, however well prepared ; and also from the observations of many physiologists, that as the excretion of urea is greatly increased after the ingestion of gelatin, it implies that the gelatin did not enter into the composition of the tissues, but was transformed in the blood, and emitted as urea.   We think that it would not be difficult to adduce arguments against these views, and particularly the facts that in our experiments gelatin caused as large an emission of carbonic acid as followed the employment of flesh meat, and also that nitrogenous matters have two actions which are useful in the economy, namely, that of forming nitrogenous tissue, and of exciting vital action.   The last action cannot be denied to gelatin, however much we may question the former ; and hence, whilst we do not attach such value to the use of gelatin as would warrant us in including that food in our scheme of dietary, we believe it to be a useful adjunct.   Iceland and Irish moss act by their mucilaginous property, and are therefore rather medicinal than dietetic substances.   We believe that the use of the new farinaceous preparation is of much value.

We do not attach importance to the employment of alcohols as articles of food under ordinary conditions, but we cannot doubt that there are circumstances in which these are called for.   If we consider that alcohol is the chief component of these fluids, we cannot employ them under the heading of these observations, viz., the increase in the supply of food, for it is impossible to affirm that it is a food in the ordinary acceptation of that term.   There are doubtless some elements in ales which supply a small amount of nutritive material, but with the conviction which we have endeavoured to establish that alcohol is not transformed in the system, we cannot extend the same remarks to spirits, and only in a very small degree will it be applicable to wines.   But we have shown[1] that indirectly this class of substances exerts a large influence over nutrition, and we purpose to describe this action when considering the mode of increasing vital action.

It will be remarked that we have not admitted tea as an article of dietary for consumptives, whilst we have recommended the use of coffee and chocolate.   The reason for this omission is the power

[1] Lancet, 1861 ; British Med. Journal, Nov. 16, 1861.

which tea possesses of increasing the action of the skin, and whilst there may be some cases in which this action would not be injurious, we believe that in the majority the tendency of it would be hurtful. Coffee and chocolate have an analogous action over the respiratory function and over nutrition, whilst they lessen rather than increase the action of the skin.

It is not unusual to recommend fish as an article of dietary in this class of cases, but we submit that in the cases in which the appetite fails somewhat, and it is desired to increase nutrition, it is much more useful to give animal flesh, with its rich juices, which offers a larger amount of nutriment in a smaller volume, and to add to it the combination of nitrogenous and hydro-carbonaceous compounds found in milk as the diluent. Without offering any very strong objection to the use of fish, we think it better to avoid it, and to supply stronger food. There are but very few cases in which the appetite refuses a moderate quantity of flesh meat, and in which the free use of milk will not form a better substitute than fish.

The two general rules to be obeyed in supplying food are, to offer the largest amount of nutriment both nitrogenous and hydro-carbonaceous in the smallest bulk, and to supply it in small quantities at short intervals.

CHAPTER XXVIII.

INCREASE THE VITAL ACTIONS.

GENERAL OBSERVATIONS.

WE have in a former part of this work shown that in many cases of early phthisis there is a small increase in the rate of pulsation and respiration, and when this is considered in connection with the emaciation which in some degree occurs, it may appear to contraindicate an increase in the vital actions, as a remedy in that disease. But we venture to affirm that this wasting of the body is no evidence of increased vital action, but rather on the contrary indicates a diminution of that vital force by which tissue is formed and the due bulk of the body is maintained, and it has long been admitted that increase in the rate of the action of the heart is *per se* evidence of feeble vital force. Hence, as the condition met with in early phthisis is truly one of lessened vital power, the increase in these actions which indicate vital power and which also maintain it, must be called for.

There are two effects of vital action which embrace all that we would affirm under this head, viz., the increase in the heat of the body, and the deposition of tissue material.

In reference to heat, we have already shown how far the waste of it may be prevented by lessening the action of the skin and the quantity of the excretions, and by this action alone the total heat in the body must be increased. But whilst it is of the first consequence to lessen the waste of heat, it is of the next importance to increase the supply of it, and then by increased production the evils of excessive waste may be altogether removed. This is effected whenever the chemico-vital changes in the body are increased, but particularly when food of whatever composition is transformed within the body.

The deposition of tissue material must also be a vital act, and to increase it considerably we must ordinarily increase the vital actions. This we conceive to be essentially the case with the nitrogenous tissues, but only partially in reference to the deposition of fat. There can be no doubt that the production of nitrogenous tissues demands the final and the highest transformation of nutritive elements, but it is not necessarily so of fat, for whilst that substance is produced within the body from other elements in food, there is no reason to suppose that fat which is taken into the body and laid up there is necessarily first transformed. Hence there are numerous instances in which increasing deposition of fat is indicative of lessening respiratory and other vital actions. Such is observed in cases of chronic bronchitis, in which it often occurs that the approach of an attack may be predicated by observing a recent increase in the deposition of fat. In phthisis, however, this increase in the quantity of fat in the body is more indicative of increase of vital action than in that of bronchitis, since it implies that the appetite for fat has been increased, and that foods containing fat in some form have been eaten more abundantly. Hence, as a general expression in cases of early phthisis, it will be correct to affirm that increased deposition of tissue elements, and of the fat contained in tissue, indicates increased vital action.

We will now proceed to consider in detail the methods whereby vital action may be ordinarily increased.

INCREASE OF APPETITE.

Whilst there is commonly a real diminution to a moderate degree in the desire for food, it is almost as common to find that caprice or unfounded belief or habit is largely concerned in that diminution. The dislike to fat and milk are patent illustrations of the fact. On inquiring into the habits of those persons who say that they have a dislike to fat, it frequently occurs that they refer only to one kind of fat, as, for example, that of meat, and the dislike may be further restricted to special kinds of fat of meat, as suet, or even the fat of beef, when that of mutton or pork will be tolerated. In this matter

there is a certain amount of fact ; for as different kinds of fat afford
different flavours, we know that persons in perfect health prefer one
kind to another ; but there is also some fiction, for it will be found
that in many cases there has been no change in the appetite, but
that the present dislike is one which has been induced by habit and
education, as is seen in families in whom it is the habit to purchase
only the leanest meat and to set the example of leaving uneaten
every small portion of fat.   So, in reference to milk, in a majority
of instances in which there is a dislike to the food, there has been
no change of recent date ; but, either in early life it was nearly
withheld, or since the period of youth its use had been almost entirely discontinued, until the absence of desire for it has been con-
strued into a distaste for it.   There are, however, a few cases in
which, with some relish for it, evil effects follow its use, as for example sickness ; but in many of these instances it will be found that
the milk is taken cold, and drunk in a tolerably large quantity at
a time, so that there has been a large accumulation of casein within
the stomach.

In nearly all the instances in which there is a declared dislike to
these two important articles of diet, it will be found that encourage-
ment and due regulation will nearly overcome the objection.   Thus,
when one kind of fat cannot be taken, another, as for example bacon, butter, suet in puddings or milk may be substituted, or it may
be eaten in smaller quantities at a time and with the addition of
starchy food.   When milk is disliked, it may be eaten when cooked
as pudding, or alone when taken hot and with bread or other farinaceous food in small quantities at a time ; and when new milk cannot be retained upon the stomach, skimmed milk may be borne.

Hence, the first duty in reference to the improvement of a defective appetite for particular kinds of food, is to ascertain how much
is due to false impressions, to habit, or to injudicious quantities, or
admixture of foods, and to regulate the habits and encourage suitable efforts to remove the distaste ; and when this has been effected,
and the mind of the patient impressed with the essential importance
of increasing the appetite for food, the whole difficulty will in many
persons have been removed.   But there will yet be many cases in
which the desire for food will still be below the requirements of the
system, and then the following rules may be applied :—

1. To allow of no improper, useless, or bulky article of food, and
   to select those kinds of food which approach to a proper dietary, and are the least distasteful to the particular patient.
2. To supply the food in small quantities at frequent intervals, so
   that the total quantity may be unconsciously increased.   The
   amount of the interval must necessarily vary with the food
   supplied ; but if the food consist chiefly of milk, the interval
   need not exceed two, or at the most, three hours.
3. To supply the food as warm as it may be comfortably eaten,

and cooked in different ways, but in those the most agreeable to the patient. The exhibition of food at a temperature
higher than that of the body is commonly practicable when
food at a temperature but little below that degree would be
rejected, and the application of the heated fluid to the stomach is fitted to increase nervous and vascular action.

Within certain limits the appetite will vary as the general vital
actions of the body vary, and hence will increase as exertion is
made or cold is applied to the body. Exertion directly causes increased vital action and increased waste, and in the ordinary course
of events increases the desire for food to supply the defect; and the
application of cold, whether by the inhalation of cool air or the application of it to the skin, acts in a similar manner, but in a much
less degree. Hence the general plan of treatment adopted in this
class of cases tends directly to increase the appetite.

The mode by which medicines increase the appetite is not very
clear. In some instances a stimulant suffices to increase the nervous
action of the stomach, or a bitter or acid constringes the mucous
coat, or an alkali removes disordered secretions ; but our knowledge
upon this point is almost exclusively empirical. We are, however,
aware by experience that condiments, carminatives, bitters, and
acids, have this influence. We have also already referred to the
stimulating influence of heat when locally employed to the stomach ;
and to this we may add the action of alcohols.

The action of alcohols as an excitant of the appetite is very well
known in India, where, with the exhaustion induced by the climate
and the low state of the vital force which occurs in the early morning, it is found almost impossible to enjoy the breakfast or the lunch
without prefacing the meal with bitter beer or some other alcoholic
compound. The like conditions do not naturally occur in this climate ; but in many cases of early phthisis the same degree of vital
exhaustion is met with, and a small quantity of ale, wine, or a little
spirit and water, when taken immediately before the meal, increases
the appetite for food. But whilst affirming the value of alcohols in
numerous instances in the condition in question, we would add that
commonly an increase of appetite would be gained without their use.

IMPROVEMENT OF THE DIGESTION.

The evidences of defective digestion are commonly a sense of fulness and load at the stomach after meals, sometimes extending to
the degree of compelling the patient to desist from eating after having taken only a few morsels ; acidity occurring in the early morning, but chiefly after meals, and a foul state of the tongue with a
disagreeable taste.

The condition in which the patient feels full after having eaten
only a very small quantity of food, appears to present a state of hyperæsthesia of the stomach. In such a case there is great liability

to vomiting if cough occur. at that period, and there is commonly
some tenderness on pressure at the epigastrium. There can be no
doubt that this condition being long continued, induces a contracted
state of the organ such as occurs when the bulk of the food is per-
manently reduced. This state is relieved by abstinence from tea,
coffee, and condiments, and by supplying food prepared with milk,
in small quantities, frequently; but if it have been long continued,
and the cavity of the stomach have been reduced in capacity, a considerable period must elapse before the stomach will exhibit the
natural tolerance to the presence of a full quantity of food at a
meal.

The most efficacious remedy in this condition is the administration
of hydrocyanic acid with an alkaline carbonate and a bitter, a short
period previous to the dinner and tea meals; and it but rarely happens that this plan of treatment, added to that which belongs to the
general treatment of the disease, fails after a few days or weeks to
allow the food to be increased in quantity, and a large quantity to be
borne during the digestive process. When, however, cases present
themselves in which this condition of the stomach is a permanent
feature, or where it is unusually intractable, it is advisable to apply
and renew blisters to the epigastrium; and it should be borne in mind
that there is no condition which so powerfully tends to obstruct the
treatment in the direction now under discussion.

The dyspepsia in which there is an excess of acidity is frequently
conjoined with that now mentioned, but in perhaps a majority of instances the acid eructations and the heartburn are more prominent
evils than the sense of fulness after meals. However the excess of
acidity may be explained, it will be found that its effect is to induce
a certain degree of irritability of the mucous membrane, and in process of time it becomes essentially connected with a diseased state
of the pharynx. In cases of heartburn the sensation is felt at the
top of the pharynx, in the part covered by tessellated epithelium, and
as we have already seen, essentially associated with the act of coughing. It is also highly probable that the inferior opening of the œsophagus into the stomach does not close, or that a certain quantity
of fluid food is retained within the cavity, as is proved by the frequent ejection of food into the upper part of the pharynx which attends the act called "heartburn." During the existence of heartburn, if a warm fluid be drunk, it causes pain in the pharynx. We
believe that in a large portion of such cases the condition complained
of is truly pharyngeal, and is not only an impediment to the reception of food, but excites cough.

It is common to find, on examining the pharynx, that portions of
food remain attached to the mucous membrane. This is the case in
that part covered by the tessellated epithelium; but whether it occurs in the lower part which possesses vibratile epithelium we cannot
tell; yet, notwithstanding the beneficial action of the ciliæ, it is very

8

probable that particles of food often remain upon the membrane. This will be the case particularly when bread or similar food is eaten alone, and the deglutition of it is not followed by a fluid. There is also reason to believe that the eructations to which we have referred have in many instances become habitual, and are due either to an unnatural action in the œsophagus, or to an abnormal formation of that organ; but, whatever may be the immediate cause, if they have been long continued, they will not readily succumb to treatment.

In this class of cases we advise that the deglutition of solid food be always accompanied by a fluid, and that fluid be drunk after the solid food has been taken. It frequently happens in health that when dry and solid food has been eaten, and particularly when it has not been well masticated, it accumulates in the lower part of the œsophagus, causes pain and perhaps hiccough, and requires a large volume of fluid to be drunk before the mass can be carried into the stomach. Hence, if the patient be subject to this accumulation, it is the more necessary that he should use sufficient fluid after the deglutition of solid food. The use of brown bread in this state is very inappropriate, since the particles of bran readily adhere to the mucous membrane, and induce irritation and acidity. We also advise the use of bread prepared with baking powder in preference to yeast, having a little excess of the alkali, since it has a less tendency to become sour, and certainly corrects acidity upon the points over which it passes. In this state, also, the use of tea, coffee, alcohols, and condiments should be interdicted, whilst antacids, either in the form of a caustic or a carbonated alkali, will be very beneficial, both at the period when the heartburn is distressing, and at other periods of the day.

We have endeavoured to connect the class of cases in which there is excess of acid secretion in the stomach and pharynx with those in which there is acid perspiration, but have not yet found any essential connection between the two conditions.

The conditions in which there is foulness of the tongue are very various, as indeed are the degrees and character of the foulness. When the tongue retains its usual size and form, and is pale, and more or less covered with a thin white layer, it may be found with any condition of dyspepsia; but the state to which we more particularly refer is one in which the tongue appears enlarged and the upper surface rounded; the papillæ enlarged and the whole organ presenting a yellow (not the ordinary pale red) tinge. There is also a thick crust over the surface, varying in thickness, but usually increasing towards the root; and there is a foul taste in the mouth, and often a foul odour in the breath. This condition we have noticed to be common in compositors and others who live in foul air and are engaged in night-work; but it is not uncommon in shoemakers and tailors, and in the poor and ill-fed. It is always accompanied by marked evidence of dyspepsia, and is usually very intractable. As we regard it rather as evidence of mal-assimilation, we shall again refer to it.

Cases of apparently pure atonic dyspepsia are not common—that is to say—conditions in which the stomach and the function of digestion simply participate in the general atony of the body; but whilst an atonic condition is observed in all the forms of dyspepsia met with in phthisis, it is commonly associated with evidence of disordered action. When, however, the atony is the leading feature, the general use of tonics, alcoholic stimulants, tea and coffee, condiments and pepsine, are the appropriate remedies.

CHAPTER XXIX.

INCREASE THE ASSIMILATION OF FOOD.

THIS, although the most important part of this branch of inquiry, is one about which but little is certainly known as to its intimate nature; it is quite clear that the food must undergo a process of final change after it has left the stomach and duodenum, and before it is deposited as tissues. It is also well known that, unless this change proceed in a due order and degree, the material which is produced is unfit for the full purposes of life, and it is termed unhealthy. This is the change which at present is hidden from our knowledge, and we are obliged as yet to be content with knowing the two extreme limits of the chain, and the causes which influence the whole process.

In the disease now under consideration there is reason to believe that this process is not healthily carried on; not so much from the production of new and unhealthy matter, as from the fact that the tissues are ill-nourished beyond what occurs in other states of the system when an equal amount of suitable food is taken. It is true that we have seen that the two anterior processes of taking and digesting food are to a certain degree in defect also; but it is probable that the deficient nutrition is still more than that defect will account for.

The circumstances which are known to have the power to increase this final transformation of food, as evidenced by the elimination of the products of transformation, are exertion, food, respiration, pulsation, temperature, and certain intimate chemical changes; and to these we will refer in their order.

EXERTION.

We have elsewhere shown that not the least amount of muscular exertion can be made without producing an increase in the quantity of air inspired, and of carbonic acid evolved. Change of posture even from lying to sitting caused in our experiments an increase of one-sixth, and to the standing posture of one-third of the quantity of air inspired; whilst walking at the rate of one, two, three, and four miles per hour, increase the quantity to 1.9, 2.76, 3.0, and 5.0 times that inspired at rest in the lying posture (page 71). The quantity of carbonic acid evolved during the exertion of walking at the rate of two and three miles was 1.85, and 2.64 times that evolved at rest in the sitting posture.

The effect over the elimination of nitrogen remains singularly mysterious. We have shown from prisoners working the tread-wheel, and Bischoff and Voit from a dog working a spit wheel, that there is scarcely any increase in the elimination of that product under the most severe exertion;[1] yet, under the theory which has of late years influenced professional opinion, the products of heat-formation were said to be eliminated by the lungs, and those of tissue-waste by the kidneys. It is, however, true, paradoxical as it may appear, that in a general sense both the observations and the theory are correct, for it has now been proved that urea is a combined product of conversion of food and degradation of tissue; and as the loss of nitrogen by the tissue during exertion is supplied by nitrogen from the food, there can be no increase in the elimination of urea from the body unless the bulk of the muscle be lessened. It must, therefore, be admitted that, with increased muscular exertion, there will be a larger emission of nitrogen from the tissue, and that the urea emitted from the body will be in a greater degree derived from the tissue than could occur in a day of rest.

In the condition of disease now under discussion, we perceive that if we increase muscular exertion, we shall increase the excretory products, and the excretory products are evidence of an increase in the metamorphosis of matter. If with this we supply sufficient and proper food, there will be both increase in the metamorphosis of the tissue, and in the final transformation of the food; and as the quantity of food transformation should be in excess of the tissue wasted, we shall cause further tissue-deposition or growth.

The due regulation of the exercise to be taken by the patient is hence of prime importance, and there are two rules which must be observed: 1st, To take as much exertion as can be borne without noticeable fatigue; and 2d, To associate the exertion with sufficient food.

In selecting the most suitable kind of exercises, we are compelled to bear in mind the strength, sex, and convenience of the patient. Athletic exercises are no doubt the best, when they are practised for a short period twice daily, and when the powers of the body are not too severely taxed. Running and jumping are suited to men, and skipping to women; and whilst the first of these sometimes

[1] Phil. Trans. 1861.

causes alarm in the minds of patients, lest hæmoptysis should be
induced, there need be no fear of its occurrence at the stage of the
disease under consideration, since the inability to breathe freely
will limit the exertion, and if any hæmoptysis should occur, it will
proceed only from the enlarged vessels of the pharynx. We feel
assured that this matter may be left to the patient, with the conviction that commonly he will make too little rather than to much
exertion. In reference to women, we attach great importance to
the practice of skipping, and direct that the rope be thrown from
before backwards, and that a considerable amount of exertion shall
be made during the ten or fifteen minutes' practice at one time.
The conventional habits of society have so limited the kinds and
degrees of exertion which females of seventeen years of age and
upwards may make, that this is almost the only one which they can
be induced to adopt as a remedial agent, and it is only after much
persuasion and explanation as to the importance of it that many will
undertake it.

But as these exercises both for males and females are presumed
to task the respiration, and will also largely determine to the skin,
they must be limited to very short periods of duration, and hence
cannot supply all that we desire. We have therefore to turn to that
of walking, as the exercise that may be the most continuously pursued, and it is highly desirable that it should be employed during
two to four hours daily. If the patient rise so as to leave the bed-
room before 8 A. M., and take a cup of milk or chocolate, with
bread and butter, it will be proper to walk in the open air briskly
for half or three-quarters of an hour before breakfast, and during
the forenoon before dinner, and again in the afternoon, from one to
two hours should be spent in exercise in the open air. The want
of strength, and the previous habits of the patient, will, in many
instances, limit the amount of exertion more narrowly than we could
desire, but it is important that the amount of exertion should approach as nearly as possible to that now recommended. It is not
however to be understood, that whilst walking during two hours,
considerable or even continuous exertion should be made during the
whole period, but such an amount of exertion should be made, and
such intervals of rest allowed, as may be practicable and agreeable
to the patient. In ordinary cases the disposition and capability for
exertion will increase by practice, and particularly if it be made in
a cheerful spirit, with a pleasant companion, in new and agreeable
scenes, and with an exhilarating atmosphere. The exertion of
walking, moreover, causes a more general use of the muscles of the
body than any other moderate exercise, and is less liable to be followed by cold than when violent exertion of particular muscles is
made, as in rowing, or when taken in closed rooms, as in various
athletic exercises. It is also capable of variation in degree.[1]

[1] We are tempted to insert here a copy of a placard which was recently exposed
in the window of a bootmaker and corncutter in one of our principal West-end

FOOD.

As food is the material to be transformed, it may at first sight appear paradoxical to look to it as an agent in its own transformation ; but whilst it is true that certain kinds of food seem to be passive in this transformation, it is equally true that there are other kinds which aid in the transformation, whilst a third class are devoted almost exclusively to the latter actions.

Amongst the passive agents we may mention the hydrocarbons, which, so far as we know, possess no power to aid in their own transformation, whilst the active agents are the nitrogenous elements. This latter fact has not been hitherto so fully admitted as it will be, since on the chemical theory, which has ruled our views of nutrition, it has only been regarded as an element of tissues, and fitted to repair the waste of tissue ; but the experiments of Lawes and Gilbert, ourself and others, have shown that the fattening properties of fodder are in proportion, not to the carbon, but to the nitrogen contained in them ; that manures containing an excess of nitrogen beyond that required to be fixed on the plant, produce better crops from the same amount of carbon in manure ; that nitrogenous foods increase the elimination of carbonic acid, and that the very large amount of nitrogen which is taken into the body beyond that which is necessary to supply waste of tissue, must be regarded as useless, if its whole duty were to supply tissue waste. Hence we have endeavoured to prove that nitrogen in food exerts the double action of promoting directly or indirectly the transformation of other food, and at the same time of supplying the wants of the nitrogenous tissues attending their degradation.

In a former part of this work, p. 144, we have urged the great importance of giving an abundant quantity of food, and particularly of the nitrogenous kind, and we have now given our reasons for that advice. It is also to be observed that there are but few instances in which nature has separated the two great classes of food ; but with the hydrocarbons has supplied the nitrogenous. This is the case with bread and flesh—the two great elements of nutrition— and nature has moreover given to us a relish for the combination of

thoroughfares, not on account of the original manner in which science is turned to commercial account, but of the talent exhibited in the composition, and the excellence of the advice! It is as follows—

"The best medicine! Two miles of oxygen three times a day. This is not only the best, but cheap and pleasant to take. It suits all ages and constitutions. It is patented by Infinite Wisdom, sealed with a signet divine. It cures cold feet, hot heads, pale faces, feeble lungs, and bad tempers. If two or three take it together, it has a still more striking effect. It has often been known to reconcile enemies, settle matrimonial quarrels, and bring reluctant parties to the state of double blessedness. This medicine never fails. Spurious compounds are found in large towns; but get into the country lanes, among green fields, or on the mountain-top, and you have it in perfection as prepared in the great laboratory of Nature.

"Before taking this medicine * * * * should be consulted on the understanding that corns, bunions, or bad nails, prevent its proper effects."

the latter with the former, and of the more highly nitrogenized with the less nitrogenized substances; and when we find the two elements separated, it is chiefly the work of man, as when he separates the starch from flour or potato, and fat from flesh.

The class of substances which, considered as food, are devoted almost exclusively to the duty of aiding in the transformation of other foods are tea, coffee, and beer. We have elsewhere[1] shown how each of these substances causes the elimination of carbon to a greater degree than it supplies that element; and hence must be the means of causing its elimination from other substances. We have not determined to which of the elements of tea and coffee this influence is due, since we have experimented only upon the substances as a whole; but in reference to beer, it is doubtless due to the nitrogenous elements, and the sugar, which they possess. It is, however, evident that these substances cannot be ranked as true foods, and that they will nourish or waste the body, not simply according to their own action, but in proportion to the amount of nutriment which is otherwise offered to the system. When the plan which we have recommended in the treatment of phthisis is pursued, and an abundance of food is supplied, these substances will aid in the nutrition of the body; but it will nevertheless be true that as milk contains so large an amount of nitrogenous matter, conjoined with the hydrocarbons, it more perfectly meets all the indications of the system than the class of substances to which we now refer.

RESPIRATION.

Respiration in its widest sense is an act which results from rather than causes vital transformation, and yet, in several important respects it modifies the transforming powers. The former fact is proved by Davy's experiments, which show that when pure oxygen was inspired there is no more chemical change induced than occurs when atmospheric air is breathed; and although we think from our own experiments that this statement will now require some modification, yet the law is established that, let the vital actions be a constant quantity, the addition of oxygen to the inspired air does not materially increase vital transformation. Hence, if we could cause an increase in the consumption of oxygen, we must begin by causing an increase in the vital actions, as by exertion and food, and in this sense the respiration obeys, and does not control, vital transformation. Allowing this statement to be true, we are led to believe that the action of the compressed air-bath must be null in this direction, for if it be in vain to offer pure oxygen in place of atmospheric air, it will be not less so to offer an increase of the quantity which is found in the air at the ordinary pressure, p. 162.

But, on the other hand, it has been proved abundantly by Vierordt and ourself, that the voluntary inspiration of an increased quantity

[1] Phil. Trans. 1859.

of air is followed by an increase in the evolution of carbon. This is primarily due to the physical action of the admixture of gases, and to the fact that the air in the central parts of the lungs is richer in carbonic acid than that found in the larger tubes, and hence deep inspiration followed by deep expiration causes a larger amount of the air, richer in carbonic acid, to be exhaled. From this it will probably follow that increased chemical change will result, for if the carbonic acid be removed from the air-cells, its place will be filled by quantities of the same gas, which will escape from the blood, and it is highly probable, that if carbonic acid be removed from the blood by any cause, it will lead to an increase of that chemical change by which it will be again supplied. Hence, whilst this train of results does not rest upon experimental proof, it is based upon physical laws which are well established.

Thus it follows that if the quantity of air expired be increased from whatever cause, there will be an increase in the vital transformation of the body; and if that be conjoined with abundant food, it will aid in the process of nutrition.

There is, however, a modifying power due to the degree of purity of the air. It has been now abundantly proved by many observers, as by De Saussure, Prof. Frankland, and Mr. Welsh, that the composition of the air at the highest attainable altitude is identically the same with that found at the level of the earth; but at the level of the earth it has been shown that there is very great diversity in the constitution of the air in town and country, and in well and ill-ventilated dwellings. Prof. Roscoe published a series of researches in the "Chemical Quarterly Journal" for 1858, in which he proved that in certain dwelling-houses, barracks, crowded schoolrooms and theatres, the quantity of carbonic acid in the atmosphere was from 1.1 to 3.3 volumes in 1000 volumes—the latter being nearly ten times the normal amount. It has also been proved that in the densely-populated parts of London the proportion of carbonic acid in the air is much increased. Now as it is known that carbonic acid depresses the vital functions, and that air cannot support life after it has obtained a certain percentage of carbonic acid, it follows that the air of densely-populated and ill-ventilated localities is less fitted to support vital transformation than the pure air of the fields and country. Dr. Angus Smith has also published some very interesting and valuable researches which establish similar facts. We may also add to this the facts, that the presence of foul air gives us an inevitable repugnance to inspire with the ordinary depth and freedom and thus lessens the effort of respiration; but the result might not appear after we had by custom become unconscious of its foulness.

But in every aspect air which is unduly loaded with carbonic acid, and which is also foul to the sense of smell, is much less fitted to promote and support vital transformation than pure air.

In the treatment of the disease in question, we have very good ground for insisting upon the patient inspiring pure air, and there-fore of his seeking the open air of the fields and the country in pre-ference to that of the bedroom or sitting-room in the crowded town.

The influence of exertion over the increase of respiration has been already pointed out, and the effect of food has also been hinted at, so that we need here only to state that the hydrocarbons—fat and starch—do not promote respiration, whilst that function is always in-creased in efficiency by nitrogenous food. Tea and coffee are the most powerful respiratory excitants amongst food, and it is singular to add, that sugar, which is a hydrocarbon, also largely increases the activity of that function.

PULSATION.

The relation of pulsation to vital transformation seems to be such that, with an unusually rapid or unusually slow pulse, there will be emaciation—the standard rate of pulsation of health in the individu-al in question being ascertained—and that in reference to rate, the normal is that which is the most compatible with the maintenance of the bulk of the tissues. It is also admitted that a certain degree of fulness of the pulse is requisite to the due performance of vital acts, for a feeble and soft pulse, whether rapid or slow, is incompatible with perfect nutrition, and, as a rule, that is the condition met with in early phthisis. A normally full pulse is therefore a circum-stance of much importance, and, whilst feebleness and rapidity of pulsation are normally associated, fulness and slowness as in the ordinary rate of pulsation are commonly found together. Hence, in treatment, the prime question seems to be, to cause an ordinary de-gree of fulness of the pulse, and in doing this the change in the rate will probably follow.

We have already referred to the conditions which modify the ful-ness of the pulse, whether it be with the *vis à tergo* or the *vis à fronte*, and will now refer only to the remedial agents to be employed to restore fulness.

The prime question, no doubt, is to increase the *vis à fronte*, whether that be by lessening the action of the skin, the kidneys, or the bowels, and thus offer greater resistance to the column of blood, and to this we have fully referred. The next question is to increase, if need be, the *vis à tergo*, by increasing the vigour of the heart, and by causing a free supply of blood to the heart through the veins of the general circulation, and through the pulmonary circuit.

The chief agents to be employed are an abundant supply of food, which, during its immediate transformation, always fills the pulse, and to administer alcohol and tonics, which tend to increase both the *vis à tergo* and the *vis à fronte*, the former by acting upon the mus-cular fibre of the heart, and the latter by lessening elimination. In this respect we think that the compressed air-bath may be of great advantage, page 159. It is evident that there will be a physical effect upon the body with the increase of the pressure, and although the pressure will be exerted both within and without the body by the air admitted within the lungs, yet it is not the less true that the pressure is increased. It will not materially affect the question whether a pressure of 100 lbs. be made upon the hand whilst it is laid flat upon a plane, or it be exerted on both sides by placing it in the jaws of a vice, for in either case there will be a degree of compression effected. So, in the compressed air-bath, we think it to be clear that the increased pressure will tend to sustain the soft structures, and particularly to support the circulation by pressure through the soft structures, both upon the surface and within the lungs. Hence, its first effect will be to give more firmness to the pulse, and it will lessen the rapidity of pulsation if the rate has been beyond that which is natural, or increase it if it have been unduly languid and feeble. Its action upon the circulation is indirect, through the intervention of the structures surrounding the vessels, and is analogous to that which, when applied to minute structures, is called tone in its influence over the capillaries.

By the courtesy of Dr. Grindrod, of Malvern, we have twice tried to determine the effect of this agent over the production of carbonic acid, and through the kindness of Dr. M'Leod, of Ben Rhydding, we have ascertained its influence over the quantity of air inspired, but at present the results are not ready for publication.

TEMPERATURE.

The influence of temperature in modifying vital transformation is very marked. When the temperature is low, as during the winter months, the excretion of carbonic acid is so largely increased that, considering the permanence of its action, the influence of this agent is probably more powerful than that of exertion. At the same period the skin is rendered less active; there is a less free distribution of blood to the surface; a large amount is retained in the central vital organs; the blood has greater capacity to retain gases, and the pulsation is somewhat slower and more vigorous. Moreover, unless the temperature be very low, the cold is favourable to exertion, and to the desire for abundant nitrogenous food. Hence, in all the points of view in which we have hitherto regarded the question of vital transformation, it is evident that cold is a most potent agent. But it is necessary that the degree of cold be such that the patient may readily tolerate it, that there be sufficient clothing and shelter to maintain the requisite temperature of the body, and abundant food to afford material for the vital transformation, and, if such be the case, there can be no doubt that the winter half year is pre-eminently suited to sustain a vigorous state of the nutritive processes in this disease.

High temperature exerts the opposite influence to that now recorded in reference to cold, since, with increase of heat, above that at which we habitually keep our dwellings, there is a rapid subsidence of the respiratory changes, and the same result also occurs with any degree of temperature, provided there be a sudden and rapid elevation of it. The pulse is commonly feeble and rapid, the blood is largely distributed to the surface, and has less capacity to hold gases in solution, the skin acts freely, the appetite for certain kinds of food fails somewhat, the tissues become relaxed, and the whole state indicates that there is a depression of the vital powers, and a diminution in the vital transformation. This condition is, however, not unfavourable to the deposition of fat in the tissues, provided the defect in the vital powers be not excessive; for we have already shown that a state in which the appetite for food is not greatly lessened, whilst the respiratory function is somewhat diminished in activity, is favourable to the storing up of fat within the system.

Hence, in cases of early phthisis, it is a prime requisite to avoid high temperature, and to permit the patient to live in an atmosphere not above sixty degrees, if it be possible to do so. This, of necessity, depends upon the period of the year, and will be the most difficult of attainment in the summer season. In the winter there is very little danger to be apprehended from the cold, if suitable precautions be taken, except in the cases in which there is inflammatory complications, or an irritable condition of the larynx, and hence no special precautions are needed, but in summer, when the temperature exceeds 65°, it is desirable that there be shelter from the sun during the heat of the day, that the day and night rooms have a free circulation of air admitted from the shady side of the house, and that the residence be in such a position as, by its elevation, northern latitude, or proximity to deep water may reduce the temperature to a medium degree. It was made clear by our own experiments that a medium temperature, such as that at which we seek to keep our houses through the year, permitted every variation in the degree of vital action according to the other conditions of season, but that as the temperature rose or fell from that central point, the effects of heat were rapidly demonstrated.[1]

CERTAIN INTIMATE CHEMICAL CHANGES.

This part of our subject is too indefinite and extensive to warrant a lengthened consideration of it on the present occasion, and we purpose only to point out one or two facts which it may be interesting to consider in the treatment of the varied conditions found in early phthisis.

It is important to bear in mind the observation which Baron Von Liebig has so often placed before us as to the importance of a due quantity of alkali in the blood, to enable that fluid to absorb the largest amount of carbonic acid. He has shown that the blood

[1] Phil. Trans. 1859.

carries carbonic acid by virtue of two qualities, viz., its property of chemical combination, and its power to hold the gas in solution, and it is evident that, in reference to actions of a rapid nature, the latter is by far the most important property. The capacity of solution varies with the nature of the fluid, and the alkaline carbonate and the phosphate of soda very greatly increase this capacity of solution in the blood. Hence the free administration of alkalies is in many cases well suited to excite or support chemical changes, and thereby to sustain vital transformation. This may possibly be one of the explanations of the beneficial action of alkalies in cases where there is marked acidity of the stomach, the perspiration, and the other excretions.

On the other hand the tissue fluids are invariably acid in their reaction, which seems to indicate that the formative process proceeds under the influence of an acid, and it is very possible that the numerous instances of early phthisis, in which the mineral acids are found to improve nutrition, may receive a part of the benefit in that direction.

M. Fernet[1] has shown that the excessive use of chloride of sodium will lessen the power of gas-absorption by the blood, since with excess of that salt in the blood the absorbing or carrying power of that fluid is lessened. This may be familiarly seen by the change of colour of black blood, which occurs on the addition of chloride of sodium, when by the disengagement of a portion of the carbonic acid the colour becomes red, and the blood is no longer enabled to retain so large an amount of carbonic acid as before. Hence the use of chloride of sodium in excess is clearly antagonistic to nutrition.

CHAPTER XXX.

REGULATE MENTAL AND BODILY LABOUR.

MENTAL LABOUR.

THE influence of mental labour over the functions of the body must be beneficial if practised within moderate limits, since without wasting the body it engages the attention, and satisfies some of the highest desires of our nature. In the abstract then, as it induces no evil, we have no remedy to offer. But when carried to excess, so that the body is constrained in posture and kept in a closed room during many hours daily, its tendency must be to exhaust the vital power, to prevent due muscular exertion, to lessen the force of the circulation, to render the skin too active, to lessen the functions of

[1] Thèse, Paris, 1858.

assimilation and digestion, and to diminish the appetite for food. Hence in this degree it is precisely fitted to induce the conditions which are observed in the disease under discussion, and demands most serious attention. There is no class of cases in which remedial agents appear to have so little influence, or in which a more decided method and long continuance of treatment are called for, as in those induced by excessive mental work, but not, as we believe, because mental labour increases the elimination of nitrogenous products, but because there has been long continued neglect of all the conditions upon which the heathfulness of the body depends. Such a state is one essentially of low vital energy.

Hence we would encourage cheerfulness of spirits and occupation of the mind in every degree compatible with the due exposure of the body to sanitary influences; and so important indeed do we consider this, that we believe it almost impossible to restore the poor man to health, who, without actual inability to labour, believes himself unfit for it, and avoids it, or the young lady who, from depression of nervous energy and bodily feebleness, is allowed to spend the day in a listless manner. A prime condition in an attempt to increase the bodily strength is the happy and moderately continuous occupation of the attention, which at the least permits the hours to pass away during which the body is regaining strength without despondency or querulous regrets; and commonly, in addition, tempts the patient to go into conditions more favourable to health.

But in the same degree do we deprecate that state of mental anxiety which renders persons at all times unhappy, leads them to shun society and the open air, and to court solitude, seclusion in the house, and distressing forebodings. Many there are suffering from early phthisis who may trace their disease to this condition, and who have been in part led into it by the adverse occurrences of life, to which all are more or less subject; and in other part by allowing anxieties to prevail over their faith and reason; and it frequently happens that the adverse circumstances continue during the disease and negative the effects of treatment. In 1,000 phthisical patients of both sexes 22.2 per cent. attributed their disease to anxiety, and the proportion was so great in women as 32.5 per cent. It is often in vain to point out the uselessness of such regrets and anxieties in reference to any attempt to remove the causes, or to show that they only aggravate the evil, and whilst kindness and courtesy may in a small degree lessen the evil, it is only as the mind can be induced to trust in him who controls all human affairs, that the calmness can be attained, which is so necessary to the use of all the means calculated to insure a return to health. Excessive anxiety, whether in reference to the prognosis of the disease or any other subject whatever, is the most formidable foe to treatment.

The effects of excessive labour are, as we have intimated, rather indirect than direct, and if they have not been too long continued, we may hope to remove them by causing the labour to cease, and by instituting the habits which we have already commended. Long continued mental labour must be opposed to the conditions upon which health of body depends.

BODILY LABOUR.

We need not insist that there is an amount of bodily labour which is not only compatible with health, but upon which health depends, and that when it is associated with a due amount of food and intervals of rest, it is our best aid in the treatment of the disease in question. The habits of mankind are in general based upon this knowledge, and the labour of the day is presumed to be proportioned to the power of the body to effect it. But there are many who from circumstances which they might control, and others from circumstances which they cannot control, allow the exertion of the body to be in excess of their power of endurance, the supply of food and the duration of rest. There are also many who labour far into or through the night, and such cannot remedy the evil by seeking repose through the day. Of these classes, we may mention the postman, the in-door-man-servant, the shopman, the night cabman, the baker, the compositor, the sempstress, the ballet-girl, and the frame-work knitter, all of whom have often come under our notice. In such cases it is necessary that the hours of labour, and the amount of walking, or other kind of exertion, be duly restricted before any attempt be made to regain the bulk and vital energy of the body. This course is especially necessary in reference to tall persons, since they demand the horizontal posture more than persons of short stature. We have elsewhere insisted upon the necessity for a periodical day of rest, and have given the physiological grounds upon which the injunction is based ; and we shall only remark here, that in the cases in question no considerable good can be effected unless this requirement be rigorously enforced.

There is another class of persons to whom it is necessary to allude, viz., such as by sedentary habits or occupations, do not make sufficient general exertion with the whole body. Such are tailors and shoemakers, in whom there is usually a deficient bodily development, and a state of very low vital power. We are accustomed in such cases to enforce violent general exercise at two periods of short duration daily, and by suitable posturing of the chest to remedy the evils attending the pursuit of the sedentary occupation. We attach the greatest importance to the pursuit of some laborious occupation or exertion in the treatment of this disease.

CHAPTER XXXI.

INCREASE INNERVATION.

THIS is either the sum of all our efforts at treatment, or it is the evidence which we seek that our efforts have been successful, precisely as we regard innervation as the cause or the consequence of vital actions. It is quite true, that if we can increase the general innervation of all the parts of the body, we shall increase the vigour of the vital process and raise the standard of health; and on the other hand we are assured that when we have increased the healthful action of the vital organs we have increased the general innervation of the body. This is indeed reasoning in a circle, but we do not think that at present our facts carry us much beyond it.

Without, therefore, entering further into the question of the origin of innervation, we may affirm that the direct tendency of all the plans which we have recommended in the treatment of this disease, is to increase innervation at the same time that they act through the various vital organs and processes of the body. In this way only do we-believe that increase of innervation is practicable; and any attempt to act primarily upon the nervous system, and through the nervous system upon the vital organs will, in the present state of knowledge, be futile. Just in proportion as the vital processes and the transformation of nutritive matter can be increased to the standard of health, and the waste of material lessened, so shall we find the evidences of increased innervation.

Dr. Churchill has proposed the use of the hypo-phosphites for a purpose very similar to that discussed in this place, and Mr. Taylor, of Liverpool, has supported his views in a paper published in the *Lancet* of October 30, *et seq.* 1861. Dr. Churchill's theory is based upon an assumption, viz.: that the excessive discharge from, or the deficient supply to, the body of oxydizable phosphorus, is the cause of phthisis, the loss of nervous force and diminution of the vital properties of the blood. We say that this is an assumption, for it is not based upon any experimental inquiries, actually showing that there is an increased excretion of phosphorus in the period preceding the occurrence of phthisis. Hence we should be justified in declining to lend an ear to Dr. Churchill's statements; but as it does not follow that his remedy is not beneficial because the grounds of his theory are defective, it will be right to try the effect of the remedy quite apart from any theory. Dr. Churchill claims that the hypo-phosphite of a base, is the best form of administering phosphorus, since it is more soluble than the phosphite or the phosphate, and also that it is capable of a higher degree of oxidation. He affirms that they increase the nervous force and promote blood formation, and he regards them as both prophylactic and curative of phthisis in every stage ; but in this he evidently affirms more than any remedy can possess, since in the advanced stage of the disease no remedy can reinstate the destroyed or useless lung. His own words are, " If, as I assert, the hypo-phosphites be the specific remedy in phthisis, because one at least of the essential conditions of that disease consists in the want or undue waste of the *oxydizable phosphorus* in the animal economy, it follows that consumption will be prevented simply by taking care to keep the system supplied with a due amount of that element. The best time for administering it is at breakfast *along with the food.*" But whilst declining to accept the whole statement, it may not be wrong to inquire if the remedy have not some virtue which may be serviceable in the treatment of the disease.

Mr. Taylor calls attention to the facts, that much impure salt is sold, that of the pure salt only 2 grains can be taken for a dose, and that it is quite necessary that even such a dose should be administered with a tonic or a carminative. He affirms that in this quantity it increases nervous and muscular force, animal heat, and the power of assimilating both nitrogenous and hydro-carbonaceous foods. But on looking carefully at his observations, it is evident that he attaches so much importance to the *adjuvans* and *corrigens*, as he terms various excellent foods and medicines, that it may be doubted if the action of the remedy could be eliminated from them.

Opposed to his view are the statements of three physicians to Hospitals for Consumption, who, after trial, have affirmed that this remedy is nearly inert. Two of these gentlemen, viz., Drs. Bennett and Quain, have prolonged its use in a few cases for several months, and whilst all ascertained that a few cases were improved during its use, and with the advantageous conditions of an hospital, there was no result which in the least indicated that the remedy excited any curative, much less, specific action. We do not, however, think, that the manner in which the inquiry has been made is such as would be admitted in physiological research, to prove the precise degree and mode of action of the substance ; for there has not been such a rigid selection of cases as would admit of parallel results, nor such elimination of attending influences as would leave the effect of this remedy evident, nor, except in a few cases, so long a duration in its use as may be demanded in the treatment of a disease which so thoroughly affects the general constitution, and which may be said to resist all treatment. We conceive the following to be the only mode by which this question could be answered :—

1. The patients to be selected should be those in the early stage of phthisis, in whom the injury done to the system is not excessive.

2. They should be treated at home, and in the conditions in which they have lived for some time previously.

3. The conditions in which they are placed should tend to health, but they ought not to be materially changed from those which have previously existed.

4. All existing causes of disease, whether within or without the body, should have been previously removed or be kept in abeyance.

5. The experiments should be continued unintermittingly during several months, and at periods of the year when there are not great atmospheric changes.

6. The aim should be to determine the effect over the elimination of important products as urea, phosphorus and water; also the amount of nitrogenous material ingested, and the proportion of that which remains in the bowel unused. At the same time the general condition of the system as to weight and innervation could be determined, and the degree of progress of the lung disease ascertained. As a basis of comparison, such inquiries should have been made upon the same person and under the same conditions during 10 days previously.

7. Six patients would be quite sufficient to prove the degree of influence of the remedy if the inquiries were thus carefully conducted.

But since we have to treat a disease which is in the long run fatal, it would be important to ascertain if the use of the hypo-phosphites were attended by results better than could be obtained from other known remedies, although they also might fail in curing the disease. Such an inquiry would be one of great difficulty, since it would imply the co-ordinate employment of other agents, the effect of which could not be isolated, but it might be pursued at least as definitely as with any other remedy. We certainly commend its employment as an adjunct to other treatment, until further experience has demonstrated its worthlessness.

Whilst being unable to affirm that the remedy is very valuable or otherwise, we must, I think, admit in general terms, that phosphorus, when combined with iron, is a good remedy in such conditions as are induced by or accompany spermatorrhœa, so frequently found in the early stage of phthisis; but that it has any specific influence over the disease such as quinine in ague, and vaccination against smallpox, as Dr. Churchill claims for it, is in the highest degree improbable, and has not been in the least proven.[1]

---

[1] Since the above was in the press, Dr. Churchill has published some papers on this subject in one of the London medical journals, and has given directions for the preparations of the salt; but we do not find that he has adduced any new proofs of the correctness of his theory.

CHAPTER XXXII.

THE LUNGS BEFORE THE DEPOSITION OF TUBERCLE,

HAVING thus concluded our remarks upon the indications for, and the details of treatment of the general system in the early stage of phthisis, we proceed to consider such local deviations from a healthy state as demand especial attention in the treatment of this disease ; and of these the most important is that of the lungs themselves.

It will be convenient to adopt the artificial arrangement of stages of the disease, and separately consider the periods before and after evidence of the deposit of tubercle.

The prime condition of the lungs in that stage which precedes the deposition of tubercle, is manifestly lessened action or lessened expansion, and consequent upon it diminished vital changes, a less free distribution of blood to the intimate structures of these organs, and a proclivity to local disease. When tubercle has been deposited, there is the presence of an extra-vascular and foreign body which must still further impede the action of the part of the lungs in which it is situate.

The deficient expansion of the lungs in its earliest condition is, no doubt, a part of the general defect of vital energy which is then existing ; for it is of common observation that when there is debility of the vital powers there is also feeble respiration ; but after a period there can be no doubt that there is a local condition induced which further enfeebles the respiratory act, and which consists in a deficient expansibility of the lungs, the result of long continued diminution of action.

Hence we have to treat both a general and a local condition, but both are so connected that the same plan of treatment is adapted to both conditions.

PROMOTE EXPANSION OF THE LUNGS.

The prime object in the treatment of this condition is (in addition to the general treatment already recommended), to produce more perfect action of the lungs—perfect in frequency and in extent of action.

For the attainment of the end here proposed we have usually to lessen the frequency of respiration, since we have seen that feebleness and frequency commonly, but not invariably, exist together ; and if we induce a deeper respiration, the duration of each act being

increased, the frequency must be in the same proportion decreased.

One of the most acute and learned physicians of our day, Sir
Henry Holland, Bart., in his classical work entitled "Medical Notes
and Reflections," has the following highly valuable remarks upon
this subject :—

"Might not more be done in practice toward the prevention of
pulmonary disease, as well as for the improvement of the general
health, by expressly exercising the organs of respiration?—that is,
by practising according to some method those actions of the body
through which the chest is alternately in part filled and emptied of
air ? Though suggestions to this effect occur in some of our best
works on Consumption, as well as in the writings of certain conti-
nental physicians, they have hitherto had less than their due influence, and the principle as such is little recognized or brought into
general application. In truth, common usage takes, for the most
part, a directly opposite course ; and, under the notion or pretext of
quiet, seeks to repress all direct exercise of this important function,
in those who are presumed to have any tendency to pulmonary disorders. Yet, on sound principle and with reasonable care, it is
certain that much may be done in this way to maintain and invigo-
rate health, even in constitutions thus disposed. Omitting some
points of controversy, particularly as to what regards the mechanical influence of respiration on the circulation through the heart and
lungs (points meriting, however, much attention from their importance), the free and equable expansion of the latter by full inspiration is beneficial ;—first, in maintaining their healthy structure by
keeping all the air passages duly open and pervious ;—secondly, in
preventing congestion in the pulmonary circulation ;—thirdly, in
providing more completely for the necessary chemical action in the
blood, by changing at each act of respiration a sufficient proportion
of the whole air contained in the lungs, and giving it more complete
access to the vascular tissues ;—all objects of great importance, and
all capable of being promoted more or less by the means in question." P. 422.

The same observer further remarks, "of actual muscular exercises
directed to this function, that of full and repeated inspiration in the
free air, is perhaps the best. The exercises which open the chest,
as it is termed, are salutary, provided they are not such in amount
as to hurry the circulation, oppress the breathing, or occasion too
large and sudden expenditure of the muscular power." Again "the
breathing, therefore, may best be exercised in these cases by full
inspiration when the body is otherwise at rest, or in slight and easy
movement. The lungs will thus be more completely filled than by
hurried respiration, and without any evil to countervail the good."
After remarking upon the beneficial influence of exercises on foot
and horseback, Sir Henry adds, "but there are cases where neither
mode of exercise is practicable ; yet, where the gentle exercise of

inspiration by voluntary effort, so as to bring more air into the lungs than is done by the common act of breathing, is advantageous even to those who are deeply under the influence of pulmonary disease." P. 428.

These observations, made many years ago, and before the precise influence of exertion over the respiration, had been determined, exhibit rare practical sagacity.

The methods by which we may increase the expansion of the lungs are four, viz., by increasing general innervation, by food, by exertion, and by deep voluntary inspirations.

BY GENERAL INNERVATION AND FOOD.

We need not here advert to the first, since we have already discussed the various plans by which innervation may be increased, and shall only affirm that the expansion of the lungs in the act of inspiration will proceed *pari passu* with the increase of innervation. The influence of foods over the expansion of the lungs has also been in part pointed out, and it is very probable that they act by a modification of the innervation of these organs. Thus we have stated elsewhere, that tea, coffee, cocoa, chicory, sugar, and nitrogenous foods increase the expansion of the lungs, and also the amount of chemical change—the former being familiarly shown by the ease and lightness of respiration, which follows the tea meal, and the latter by the increase in the carbonic acid evolved. But the amount of the increase of expansion due to their influences is but small—seldom exceeding 10 cubic inches at each inspiration, and as a mechanical action it cannot be regarded as very important.

BY EXERTION.

The effect of exertion is very considerable according to the degree of it. During ordinary quiet respiration we inspire from 35 to 45 cubic inches at each act, but when we run at full speed, or on working the tread-wheel, the quantity is increased to upwards of 100 cubic inches at each inspiration, and the inspirations are increased from 12 to upwards of 20 per minute, until the increase of the pace prevents the amount of lung action which is necessary to accompany it, or until the duration of the more moderate pace has wearied the muscles both of the general system and of the chest. The difference in the amount of expansion requisite to admit 40 and 100 cubic inches of air is very great, and the amount of vital force exerted to make the greater effort, and to perform it with a speed $2\frac{1}{2}$ times as great at each inspiration, and with twice as many inspirations in a given time, must be greatly increased. Hence we have in this degree of exertion a most powerful agent for the purpose in hand. More moderate degrees of exertion are attended by less increase of respiratory action, but yet cause an increase of very great value. Thus, in walking at the rate of 1, 2, 3, and 4 miles per hour, the depth of inspiration was increased in our experiments to 52 C. I., 60 C. I., 75 C. I., and 91 C. I. at each inspiration, and the frequency of respiration was 18, 18½, 22, and 25 per minute. The sauntering pace of two miles per hour causes an expansion of the lungs, and a rate of respiration of ½ more than that observed at rest, and is far more powerful than we are accustomed to believe. When, therefore, the patient is enabled to take a moderate amount of exercise, we must admit that in doing so he is placed in very good circumstances to produce the mechanical as well as the chemical effect which we desire; but if, in addition, running, jumping, or skipping be performed for short periods, the effect is greatly increased. He should also be informed of the object which the medical adviser has in view, and reminded that it is desired to produce complete expansion of the chest. He should endeavour, during the exertion, to breathe lightly and freely, and with as much depth of inspiration as may be convenient to him.

In numerous cases it will be necessary to encourage the efforts of the patient to the performance of any required degree of exertion ; for it is not infrequent to meet with those who, from a sense of weakness, dyspnœa, and pleurodynia on exertion, or defect in the previous habits, believe themselves unable to make so much exertion as is required. To this end it is advisable that such exercises be selected as are convenient to the patient, and that the amount be gradually increased ; but in whatever degree it may be made, it must be carefully limited in time.   Any degree which induces true fatigue is in excess, but by judicious management this degree may be gradually increased without inducing a sense of fatigue.   In a case of early phthisis we advised, in addition to other exercises, the use of the skipping-rope within doors, in the middle of October, and at that time it was found that she was unable to skip more than three times without inducing so much pleurodynia and dyspnœa as to compel her to rest ; but, by careful continuance twice a day, she was able in the course of a month to skip more than 100 times without resting and without fatigue.   In a similar manner, ladies who have not been accustomed to walk one mile per day out of doors may, by gradual increase, and the use of a hand-chair when tired, become able to walk 5 or 6 miles daily with comfort.

BY DEEP VOLUNTARY INSPIRATION.

Considering the duration of exertion and the aptitude which all have for it, it is probable that we possess no agent which is equally powerful for the purpose now under discussion ; but in reference to short periods of action, we find deep voluntary respirations yet more efficacious.

These are performed by inducing the patient to breathe as deeply as the lungs will allow, with the view of expanding the chest to the utmost possible limits. To this we attach the greatest importance, and having advocated it for some years past, we are much gratified to find that so distinguished a physician in diseases of the chest as M. Piorry has arrived at the same views, and recommends this plan of treatment as unreservedly as we do, and with the higher authority which attaches to his name and fame. It is true that the object sought by M. Piorry and ourself does not appear to be identical, since his primary aim seems to be, the difficult and important one of producing the resorption of deposits, and in this he affirms that he succeeds; whilst our chief aim is to increase the expansibility or patency of the lungs, and thus increase chemical change and prevent the occurrence of deposits; but there is such an analogy between these two objects, that the treatment of each may be regarded as practically the same.

The production of this complete expansion of the chest is oftentimes a circumstance of extreme difficulty, and sometimes it cannot be effected; but the difficulty lies not in any impediment to the entrance of the air, but in the defect of muscular power to expand the chest, or in the impossibility of inducing the patient to comprehend the method by which it is to be effected. Hence, however great the difficulty, it lessens by practice, if the practice be carefully and intelligently made.

The plan which we adopt is as follows:—

The patient is placed in the sitting or standing posture, with the trunk erect, the shoulders drawn downward and backward, and the chest thrown forwards. The mouth is then kept a little open, and the patient is directed to inhale gently whilst he very evenly expands the chest to its utmost limits; and at the end of the inspiration he is directed to make increased effort, and then to retain the chest in its expanded state for two or three seconds before expiration is commenced. If the mouth be shut, the nostrils cannot admit the volume of air with sufficient freedom; and if, instead of an even and somewhat gentle inspiration, the air is drawn in quickly and forcibly, like suddenly snatching asunder the handles of a pair of bellows, it is impossible for the lungs to become perfectly expanded. If, at the end of the inspiration, there be not increased effort made, the mechanical act of distension is materially lessened, and the good which is effected is imperfect; whilst there is a manifest advantage in keeping the lungs fully expanded for a few moments, and afterwards in preventing a collapse of the chest by a sudden and rapid expiration. The posturing of the chest is also important, not only by inducing that position in which the cavity may be most completely enlarged, but, by placing the relaxed and elongated pectoral muscles upon the stretch, and holding the shoulders firmly backward, the greatest amount of muscular power may be obtained.

There are two of these conditions which it is very difficult to fulfil, viz., the prevention of a rapid and gasping inspiration, and the final effort at the end of inspiration to effect the complete dis-

tension of the lungs.   The former is more common in cases where
the respiration is short, and the person is nervous and defective in
readiness of apprehension, and in such cases is very difficult of
attainment; whilst the latter is chiefly associated with much atonicity of the muscular system, and in the most intelligent and painstaking person is only perfect after long practice.   Its increase is,
however, a good measure of the improvement of the patient.

On deep inspiration we find that the apex of the lung is not filled
until the very end of inspiration, and we have explained this at page
122, by the common direction of the Bronchi, which carries the
current downwards, and also by the great extent and direction of
motion of the lower ribs, so that whilst in inspiration the air is admitted into all permeable parts of the lung, the lower part is first
filled by voluntary effort, and then the upper.   Hence, for various
reasons, we see the importance of the effort to inspire at the very
end of the act of inspiration, with a view to cause the complete expansion of the apices of the lungs.

We have found it always necessary to have the chest uncovered,
and to watch carefully the movements of the parts during this
procedure, so as to appreciate any defect in the performance; and
moreover, it is commonly needful that the physician should show
the action upon himself.   It is needless to state that it is an easy
process to those who can do it; but as its entire value rests upon
the degree of perfection with which it can be effected, it demands
that the physician be enabled from time to time to inspect the movements and correct their defects.

It is also evident that deep respirations cannot be continuous,
since their duration is incompatible with the ordinary rapidity of
respiration, and therefore we direct that after each complete expansion of the chest there be one or two ordinary inspirations effected,
and that with these alternations the practice be continued for ten
minutes at a time, and be renewed once or twice in the day.   It may
also be performed in the house, if the air be pure; or out of doors
if the air be warm.

It is a method of treatment which is attended with a rapid increase in the expansibility of the chest, so much so that the practice
of a few weeks will cause the front of the chest below the clavicles
to advance and project on deep inspiration, when before it was flattened.   It has also the advantage of amusing the patient, and of
finding an occupation for the mind in the search for health; and any
other general and local treatment may be adopted at the same time.

If this complete expansion of the chest be daily effected, and at
the same time the vital actions of the whole body be invigorated,
and the various plans to which we have referred have been effected,
we affirm that if tubercle be not already deposited, it is fitted to prevent its deposition; and if already existing in a small degree, it will
in all probability prevent its increase, and the parts of the lungs not
thus occupied will regain their normal condition.   This improve-

ment, or cure, will of course be dependent for its continuance upon the maintenance of a due degree of vigour of system, and will pass away if at any time the conditions which first led to it shall be renewed.

Hence we consider that up to the point under discussion, phthisis is as curable as any other condition of an organ in which an equal deterioration in the function or structure has occurred.

CHAPTER XXXIII.

THE LUNGS AFTER THE DEPOSITION OF TUBERCLE.

ORDINARY LIMITS OF REMEDIABLE CONDITIONS.

As we have limited ourselves to a consideration only of those conditions in which phthisis is a remediable disease, it is necessary here to determine the amount of disease which we believe to be remediable. This is a task of no ordinary difficulty, for, on the one hand, the term may be held to require that all the conditions of the disease shall be removed, and, on the other, that we shall be able rigorously to limit the extent of the disease. As to the former we may remark, that we shall fulfil all that can be desired, if in many cases every trace of disease be removed, and if in others we can arrest the disease so that there shall be no longer any danger of its progressing; and as to the latter, we shall be satisfied to confine ourselves to such conditions as are commonly determinable on the most careful examination.

We think, therefore, that after tubercle has been deposited, the case is remediable under the following conditions:—

1. When the amount of tubercle is small, its site capable of careful definition, and the other parts of the lung free from disease.
2. When the deposit is found in only one lung, even if it have proceeded to a somewhat greater extent.
3. When the vital powers of the general system are not greatly depressed, and where there is no complicating disease.
4. When the progress of the deposition has not been rapid.
5. In cases where there is a small isolated cavity surrounded by healthy lung, without pleuritic adhesion, and one lung quite sound. When the cavity is empty, and has remained so for some time, the case is more hopeful.
6. When the patient can and will adopt all the plans which are necessary for his restoration to health.

Such are the conditions in which there may be hope of restoration to health, and either of true cure, or of complete arrest of the disease so long as the patient lives under healthful conditions; but we do not wish to intimate that, occasionally, arrest may not occur in a more advanced state of the disease. We shall again refer to this subject under the head of Prognosis.

DEEP VOLUNTARY INSPIRATION.

In each of the above conditions we still advise the most careful use of the method of deep voluntary inspirations, with a view to maintain the patency and vital activity of all the parts of the lung at present free from disease, for in so doing it is highly probable that the further progress of the disease will become impracticable.

REMOVAL OF TUBERCLE.

The aim, in reference to the tubercle deposited, must be either to promote its removal, or to isolate it, and induce the cretaceous degeneration.

In reference to the removal of tubercle we do not think that anything can be done to promote it by the expectoration, since it may be doubted as to how far any expectorant has effect upon the air-cells themselves, however much it may have upon the bronchial mucous membrane; and as a rule we should discountenance the use of expectorants at that period, lest they should tend to induce a state of congestion and irritation of the tissues. For the same reason we do not advise the employment of inhalations which have an irritating tendency. The efforts at removal must certainly be directed to the absorbents by which the material may be disintegrated and altogether removed, or the fluid parts removed and the solids left in a state to which we shall presently refer. For this purpose it seems to be necessary that the tubercle should either have been recently deposited and have undergone no secondary changes, in which case the promotion of its absorption is the direct road to the cure; or after having been long deposited in small quantities only, it has degenerated, and finally softened without inflammatory action, in which case the capability of being absorbed has occurred as a secondary result. It is, however, to the former that we particularly refer at present as the condition in which the aim may reasonably be to cause its removal by absorption.

We have already referred to the opinion of M. Piorry, that the voluntary and deep inflation of the lungs directly tends to promote the absorption of deposited matter. This is highly probable, both from the fact that such treatment directly tends to the increase of vital action, and also from the pressure which it mechanically affords, and which in certain conditions is known to be favourable to the absorption of fluids. Hence the plan already recommended receives another sanction.

Of the medicinal agents to be employed for this purpose, we at-

9

tach great value to the administration of iodine in small doses, and
of all forms that of the iodide of iron has appeared to us to be the
most efficacious.   The syrup is an agreeable preparation, but the
iodide of iron in pills is, we think, to be preferred for adults, and of
this 2 grs. should be taken thrice a day, for a period of six or eight
weeks without intermission.   We have not found the use of iodide
of potassium so fitting in these cases as in those of deposits from
chronic pneumonia, and generally because the system does not gain
strength under its use, and does not well bear it.   It is possible that
in some cases the inhalation of iodine may also be serviceable, but
generally its action as a local irritant, and particularly where the
fauces exhibit much irritability, has prevented our employing it extensively.   The application of the iodine paint to the walls of the
chest cannot, we think, act in this manner with any degree of
certainty, since the anatomical disconnection of the parts renders
the action upon the lung-structures almost impossible.   We need
not here advert to the fact, that the tendency of all the remedies
previously advised is to promote this absorption, since they tend to
improve the tone of all the vital powers.

We have already referred to the conditions of tubercle in which
this action may be looked for, but it is necessary further to add,
that, in a majority of the cases, it is probable that only the fluid and
the unorganized animal parts will be removed, and that there will
remain whatever is truly solid, whether in the horny state to which
Laennec and his school often referred, or in the mineral matter
which occurs with secondary changes.

ISOLATION OF TUBERCLE.

This result is almost as valuable as the former, for although the
material remains, it is placed in circumstances which are comparatively harmless.

This is effected when, after a small amount of deposition, the
further progress of the disease is arrested; for in nearly all such
states the tubercle, in process of time, puts on secondary changes
which tend to its permanent isolation.   This end is promoted by
whatever improves the general health, but particularly by the full
inflation of the lungs, the first by tending to remove the general,
and the second the local conditions upon which the deposit depends.
The latter remedy acts no doubt both by maintaining the patency
of such cells as are free, or nearly so, from the deposit, and by promoting the closure of those which are nearly filled by it, for as the
healthy air vesicles which surround a small mass in which the deposit has occurred are fully distended, they must cover and press
upon those which are incapable of inflation, and thus soon cut off
any communication between the latter and the external atmosphere.
This we believe to be a most important effect of the agent in question, and a mode whereby the isolation of the tubercle is most readily

effected. It is also to be borne in mind that the lobular arrangement of the lung aids this result, since by it small aggregations of
air-cells are inclosed in an inexpansible membrane, and connected
with the air by one minute ramifying tube only, which after a period
may become impervious.

Hence there can be no doubt that the cases of isolated calcareous
tubercle are commonly cases of true arrest and cure, but calcareous
tubercle is very frequently found in the sputa of persons in whom,
if there have been arrest, it has been only temporary, and who suffer from destruction of the lung tissue of greater or less importance.

ISOLATION AND POSSIBLY CLOSURE OF A CAVITY.

From the period of Bayle it has been noted that puckered conditions of the lungs have been found which more or less resemble a
cicatrix, and that on carefully cuttting into it the structures have
been found tough and solid, and sometimes resembling cartilage. These
were, therefore, regarded as evidences of the prior existence of an
abscess or a vomica which had gone through its course of destructive
excavation, followed by emptying and contraction, and had ended by
simply inducing the loss of a large number of air-cells. Such is a
ready, and probably in many cases a true explanation of the appear-
ances, and hence we find a certain amount of warrant for the belief
that cavities may entirely disappear. Moreover, we find in practice
a certain small number of cases in which there is a small and isolated
cavity at the apex of the lung, which readily empties itself, does not
tend to increase, and in which there is no further deposition of
tubercle, whilst watched over a period of months or one or two years.
There are also other instances in which, with more extensive mischief,
we find evidences of a dry cavity which has existed for years, and
in which there has been little or no accumulation of secretion.
Such may add to the presumption of cure, but doubtless they are
rare when compared with the mass of cases, and must be included
in a category of curable conditions with a certain reservation.

When, however, we find a small isolated cavity without tendency
to increase, and without further tuberculous deposition, our aim
should doubtless be to induce its closure. How may this be effected?

Those cavities appear the most fitted for this process which are
small, and have not any quantity of infiltrated tubercle in the tissues
which bound them—that is to say, such as have thin and still elastic
sides. It has been presumed that closure occurs partly by the
filling up of the cavity with exudations, and partly by the collapse
of the sides. The former is scarcely possible in any case in which
the cavity is of size to deserve the name, both from the impossibility
of accounting for the deposition of layer within layer more and
more distant from the bloodvessels, and from the fact that the
remains of cavities exhibit the marks of compressed tissues rather
than those of accumulated foreign material. The collapse of the

sides of the cavity of the nature above mentioned must certainly occur, and if it be placed in the apex of the lung, and be free from pleuritic adhesion, the upper part will fall downwards so as to tend to obliterate it from above.

In reference to this mode of closure voluntary inflation of the lung is very useful, for as the adjoining cells become fully expanded, they must press upon the sides of the cavity, and as there will be less resistance in that than in other directions, the air-cells will the more readily tend to expand at the superficies of the cavity. It may be objected that in such conditions the forcible expansion of the lungs will be likely to induce hæmoptysis, but in the course of extensive experience we have not found that result, and, indeed, when we recollect how much less force is used in the expansion of the lungs by the inhalation of air with the trachea open than by the effort of coughing, when with the trachea closed there is violent and sudden compression of the air from below, so as to forcibly expand the air-cells of the upper and the least resisting parts of the lungs— we shall see that there is much less probability of hæmoptysis occurring with this act than with coughing. It may also be objected that an emphysematous condition of the air-cells abutting upon the sides of the cavity may occur by forcible inspiration, and it is possible that both by this act and by coughing this may occasionally follow, yet it does not complicate the case adversely, but rather favourably, for in so doing it must tend further to lessen the cavity.

To these various acts we must add that of the natural contractibility of the yellow elastic tissue of the lung, and of the membrane lining the cavity when the cavity remains empty, and whilst we do not think that this would greatly tend to advance the required end by itself, we must admit that it is an important condition with which the other agents may act. It is also clearly an essential preliminary condition that the cavity either be empty or have a free outlet for all secretions.

COLLAPSE OF THE AIR-CELLS.

Having thus treated of the relation existing between the puckered' cicatrices found on the lungs and the closure of cavities, we think it needful to add that such appearance would be readily accounted for by mere collapse of a mass of air-cells, by which a depression in the lung would occur, and the tissues be compressed together and lose their configuration. That such a state should occasionally occur must be admitted, since it only needs that the minute bronchial tubes should become impervious, as by local pressure of internal deposits, after which the air would become absorbed, the cells would collapse, and the adjoining cells would partly fill the space thus vacated. That it does often occur in the lungs of infants is well known. We would therefore venture to suggest that such cicatrices cannot be accepted as indisputable evidence of the pre-existence of a cavity.

CHAPTER XXXIV.

THE THROAT.

WE have intimated that there are two principal conditions of disease of the throat met with in numerous cases, in the early stage of phthisis, and that they are important, less in themselves than from the cough which they occasion. The two conditions may be termed anæmic and congestive respectively.

In the anæmic throat the leading indication, as a local condition, is to lessen the hyperæsthesia, which is commonly present; and the most satisfactory remedies are the strong solution of nitrate of silver, or an admixture of chloroform and neat's-foot or cod-liver oil.   In both applications it is better to use a large camel's-hair brush, quite as large as the end of the little finger.   The patient should be seated before a light, and the tongue being carefully depressed by the spatula, whilst the patient is breathing through the mouth, the brush having been dipped in the application and drained a little upon the edge of the vessel, must be well swept round the fauces, so as to apply the solution to the posterior wall of the pharynx, as low down as the epiglottis.   The only difficulty in this process is to induce the patient to breathe through the mouth (not through the nose) and thus raise the velum palati from the tongue, and to breathe with freedom and ease, so as to prevent the act of vomiting and allow time for the careful application of the remedy.

There is with either remedy a certain amount of choking induced by the approximation of the epiglottis to the pharynx from reflex action, but it is never alarming or long-continued with the chloroform.   In reference to the application of the nitrate of silver, however, we have seen the most alarming spasm, and so severe a sense of choking as to prevent inspiration, and so continued as to induce discoloration of the face and great terror to the patient.   After half a minute, perhaps, this passes away, and commonly at the moment when there is an eructation of flatus which had been pent up in the contracted œsophagus, when the larynx and pharynx were temporarily closed.   We have never met with any untoward results, but the danger appears imminent in some of those cases in which the hyperæsthesia is considerable, and hence we commonly, on the first occasion, apply the caustic to the tonsils and uvula only, where there is not the power to excite the reflex movement which closes the larynx and pharynx.   If this application be well borne, the next step is to apply the solution sparingly to a part of the posterior wall of the pharynx; and if that should be tolerated, it may be safely applied over the whole surface of the pharynx on the next occasion.

In this condition of the throat, notwithstanding the general blood-lessness of the mucous membrane, there are commonly a few large and superficial veins traversing the surface from above downwards, and from which the blood in hæmoptysis often proceeds. It is apparently of importance to cause contraction of these vessels, and this will be effected by the application of the solution of caustic, or, failing that, by a touch of the solid caustic in some spot in the course of the vessels.

This is the condition of the throat which, *par excellence*, belongs to phthisis, and whilst the state of congestion or suffusion is also met with, it is much more rare, and is commonly due to conditions apart from phthisis. Thus it may oftentimes be traced to the use of neat ardent spirits, to the free indulgence in tobacco, and particularly when used with a foul pipe, or to the inhalation of irritating fumes, as those of charcoal burnt in a stove without free ventilation, or on the open hearth in certain manufactures, or those proceeding from the combustion of impure gas in badly-ventilated rooms. Hence the treatment of it is almost apart from phthisis; but we have found the application of chloroform and oil, or the frequent use of warm suet and milk in small quantities, or the taking of cod-liver oil alone, or made into an emulsion, with an alkali, the best remedies. It is also requisite to remove internal obstructions to the circulation by purgatives or alteratives, or to determine to the skin, as the case may require; and as there is usually tenderness, on pressure, over some part of the throat, it is very useful to apply, and re-apply, small blisters as near to the part affected as possible. When there is much relaxation of the throat, or the colour of the mucous membrane is deepened by the duration of the disease, it frequently happens that the application of the strong solution of caustic is attended with benefit; but we do not advise it in the earlier stage, or when there is the appearance of acute desquamation of the epithelium.

In both conditions of the throat it is well to employ such remedies as by locally covering the membrane will, for a time, prevent the immediate contact of the air; such are oily and alkaline emulsions, or gelatinous, albuminous, or mucilaginous fluids, and it will also do good service if such a sedative as morphia, mixed with thick mist. acaciæ or thick syrup of poppies, be drank very slowly and taken in small quantities, so that it may have an immediate action upon the mucous surface. It is also true that sedatives and narcotics, when taken in pills, or other form, so that they cannot exert a local action as they pass over the sensitive surfaces, yet lessen the sensibility through the general system; but we submit that this is a very circuitous mode of action, and very liable to disturb other parts which do not need the sedative influence. It is certainly better to administer the remedy in such a form that it may act directly upon the part affected, and be administered in small quantities and frequently. We venture, also, to affirm that cod-liver oil, when it acts beneficially, often does so by the local action upon the throat, producing the soothing effect, and relieving the cough, to which so many patients ascribe its utility.

CHAPTER XXXV.

HÆMOPTYSIS.

THE treatment of hæmoptysis in phthisis always demands careful consideration and preliminary investigation, and the ordinary habit of repressing it by styptics is often fraught with much danger.

In the majority of cases the amount of bleeding is so small as not to attract much attention, and in such any special treatment for its arrest would be unnecessary; but even in other instances in which it is more profuse, its importance really lies in indicating a condition of the circulating system, or some other part of the body, than any mischief to which it may give rise.

The first duty on the occurrence of hæmoptysis is to examine the chest and the fauces. If there be evidences of congestion of the lungs as a whole, such as may be proved by diminished resonance and lessened respiration, with a sense of constriction or dyspnœa, and with more or less disturbance of the general system, or if there be similar evidences restricted to a part of the lung, whether at the base or apex, and shown more particularly after a certain amount of effusion has occurred by crepitation or indistinct moist rales, the proper course will be to relieve the bowels, to determine to the skin, and to enforce the maintenance of the horizontal posture. Unless the discharge be considerable, it is not advisable to employ cold, either by ice or cold and comfortless food, or exposure to cold air, since the aim is not repressent, but derivative. The use of hot foot-baths and saline diaphoretics, the application of blisters between the shoulders, or the use of the croton oil liniment to a large part of the chest, will be the proper course; and unless active inflammation should follow, the hemorrhage will soon be arrested.

When there is evidence of inflammatory action the case assumes a character which cannot be treated of here, and the severity of the antiphlogistic regimen must depend upon the circumstances of the case.

When the hemorrhage can be traced from enlarged vessels in the pharynx, the case may be left to general treatment, unless it be urgent, when the local application of a solution of nitrate of silver (30 grs. to an ounce) by the aid of a large camel's hair brush, or of the solid caustic, to any particular vessels which may be seen, will be proper. The use of styptic gargles, as those of alum, borax, and tincture of the sesquichloride of iron diluted, with water, may be employed in continuance of treatment.

There are, however, many instances in which it is necessary to act upon the blood, either from the condition of that fluid, or the fact of the hemorrhage being probably a transudation through the membrane, or from a vessel bursting into a cavity in the lungs beyond our reach. In all of these cases we have found great benefit from the use of an aqueous or a spirituous solution of the perchloride of iron, made in the proportion of 5 drachms of the salt to 6 ounces of water or proof spirit, and given in doses of twenty to thirty drops in water six times a day. Warren's styptic, made by the addition of 2 drachms of turpentine and alcohol each to 5 drachms acidi sulph. fort., and then filtered through sand, is also a most efficient remedy, and the dose may be 15 to 30 drops in water. The employment of 1 scruple to half-drachm doses of turpentine in mucilage is an old and very valuable remedy, and to these may be added the employment of gallic, tannic, and dilute sulphuric acids, in doses of 8 grains of the two former, or 1 scruple to half-drachm of the latter. The use of ice gradually dissolved in the mouth is very valuable.

We meet also occasionally with cases in which the hæmoptysis is clearly associated with the menstrual function, and is erroneously considered vicarious. In such cases the menses are greatly reduced in quantity, and not infrequently changed in quality, and the hæmoptysis occurs either at the period of their occurrence, or at the usual monthly period when they are absent. We have seen numerous instances of the former, in which there was much uneasiness at the stomach for two or three days preceding, and on the day of the occurrence of the insufficient menstrual discharge, so that the cases assumed rather the features of ulceration of the stomach, until the periodicity and the relation to the menses had been clearly established. It is always very difficult to decide upon the direct plan of treatment in these cases, since the discharge gives no relief, is attended by suffering, and occurs in enfeebled persons, and yet there is no indication which would justify the employment of styptics. The only safe plan is to enforce the horizontal posture, to give mild diluents as food, to regulate the general functions, to use the mustard foot-baths, and to apply a mustard-plaster to the lumbar region of the spine.

Hence, on a review of this subject, we venture to affirm the following general rules :—

1. That commonly the hæmoptysis is unimportant, except as indicating a condition of the general system, or of the pharynx or of some portions of the lung.

2. That its repression by direct means is often highly prejudicial, and tends to further advance in the disease of the lungs, and that in no case is it justifiable without a careful examination of those organs,

3. That ordinarily the plan of treatment is tonic and derivative.

CHAPTER XXXVI.

MUSCULAR PAINS.

THE myalgia to which we have already referred as a pre-existent and concomitant condition of early phthisis, is that of the muscles about the chest, some of which are connected simply with the arm, and others with the acts of inspiration and expiration. The former induce distress, and therefore demand alleviation, but the latter limit the respiratory motions, and thereby all the vital and mechanical actions which attend them, and more or less induce danger to health. The indications for treatment are various, and include the removal of any mechanical or vital cause, the improvement of the general tone of the system, and the use of local derivatives.

As the weight of the arm is borne by the muscles attached to the neighbourhood of the shoulder, there is a constant tendency in these muscles to the condition known as weariness, and in order to avert or relieve this, we direct that the arm be artificially supported, as when leaning upon a table. But there are engagements as those of a sempstress, in which, whilst one arm may be thus supported, the other must remain free for motion, and hence there is a cause of inequality of muscular effort, and of suffering on one side only. This will illustrate numerous conditions in which muscular pains arise, and the first duty is to limit the period when the muscles of the shoulder must bear the weight of the arm, and to render the support equable on both sides. This will often suffice to remove the pain, but if it should fail, or if it cannot be effected, the most efficient remedy is artificial support by plasters. We do not find that the nature of the plaster is material, since we believe it to have a mechanical effect only, but it is requisite that it be made upon a substantial material, as very thick calico or leather, that it be much larger than the extent of the pain, that it fit and stick very closely, and be renewed as often as the support which it affords fails. We cannot deny, in reference to its mode of action, that there is also besides the mechanical support a certain degree of irritation induced, an excitement of the sweat ducts, and a most potent protection against the accession of cold air, and it is possible that one or all of these may be of some value in the action of plasters under all conditions. Indeed, in reference to the latter action, we frequently advise the use of several plasters when there is indistinct pain and liability to cold of the front or back of the chest, and believe them to be most efficient safeguards. The employment of stimulating liniments in this condition has also been commended, but although we have occasionally seen great relief afforded by the use of strong turpentine or ammoniacal liniments, we have been much more frequently disappointed than when calefacient, belladonna, opium, or other plasters have been applied, and since both cannot be employed at once, we are required to choose between them.

In the numerous cases in which the pain is restricted to a small surface, and is very acute, we believe that no remedy is equal to blisters. One application of the blister commonly removes the pain, but occasionally cases occur in which it is necessary to renew the application several times. It may perhaps be an open question as to whether the iodine paint or the Spanish flies is the best mode of causing a denuded surface, and, whilst admitting that they are equally good in many cases, we prefer the blister when the pain is very localized and very acute, and the iodine when the pain is severe but less acute, and is experienced immediately beneath the clavicle, where the figure of the chest is uneven and not well adapted for the application of blisters. When the iodine paint is freely used, the pain to which it gives rise is greater than occurs with blisters, and it produces a sore, secreting a pus, and sometimes not easily healed ; but when it is lightly applied, the degree of irritation may be more carefully graduated than can be effected with a blister. The croton oil liniment is also a valuable agent, but seldom so trustworthy as a blister in the treatment of myalgia, yet when the pain is widely distributed over the chest, it is more convenient to use this more general remedy than the strictly localized blister. The croton oil often causes irritation in the eyes, and it frequently happens that the eruption extends to parts which apparently have not been rubbed with the oil. There is also much diversity in the effect produced upon the different skins, so that occasionally a single application will cause great irritation, whilst commonly three applications must be made daily for two or three days before the desired effect is produced. When we order this application, we direct it to be employed thrice a day, and continued with short periods of intermission for some weeks, unless the pain should have in the meantime passed away. There are some cases in which the myalgia has a rheumatic character, although they are few in which this can be ascertained with certainty. The history of the case is the best guide, but in addition the intractable character of the pain under the ordinary treatment may sometimes aid us. In such cases we find that the exhibition of colchicum in the form of the acetic extract, or the powdered root conjoined with Dover's powder, is the best remedy, in addition to the external application already advised.

In the intractable cases which are connected with spermatorrhœa, we have found the improvement of innervation and of the bodily functions in general, with the use of cold bathing and occasional blistering, to be the most efficacious. It is in such cases that the phosphate of iron sometimes produces marvellous benefit.

CHAPTER XXXVII.

CATEGORICAL STATEMENT OF THE WHOLE PLAN OF TREATMENT.

WE purpose in this chapter to state, in as few words as possible, and without comment, the details of treatment which are suited to a case in the early stage of phthisis, and which have been already discussed at length; but it will be understood, *in limine*, that any general plan will require to be modified in reference to the treatment of individual cases, as certain conditions of the system are more or less pronounced in each case.

FOOD.

The patient should take from two to three pints of milk daily, prepared (and we also add *thickened*) with chocolate, arrowroot, flour. gluten semola, oatmeal, or bread, or made with eggs, &c., into puddings. In cases where new milk does not agree, skimmed milk may be in part supplied, and then, if fats be tolerated, half an ounce of suet, cut finely, should be well boiled in each pint of milk, and taken quite warm. The milk should be eaten in somewhat small quantities, say half a pint at a time; one quantity is to be taken immediately on the patient awaking in the morning, others at breakfast and supper, the milk pudding for dinner, and chocolate or coffee may be added to the milk which is taken at breakfast and tea. Food should further be taken at intervals of from two to three hours, and the dinner should be supplied soon after midday. Half a pint of good soup, with bread, may be taken between breakfast and dinner, and, if fats are not disliked, it would be better to prepare the soup from ox .heads or shins, so as to supply both oil and jelly in addition to the juices of the meat, and the whole should be well thickened with groats or corn flour. Eggs, bacon, or meat should be taken at breakfast, and abundance of fresh meat at dinner. with soup, pudding, and a moderate quantity of fresh vegetables, French beans, and bread. The meat should be of the richest quality, and have at least one-third of its weight of fat. If the patient like salad oil, it may be eaten as freely as possible. A small quantity of cheese should be added to the dinner. An egg should be taken at the tea meal and also at supper when milk is not taken. There should also be a cup of milk and bread and butter placed at the bedside of the patient, and eaten, if possible, during the night. Beer or wine may be taken at dinner, and once or twice at other periods of the day, if it be found to agree with the system, and the dose be so moderated that it may not in the least affect the head, or cause heaviness in, and indisposition to move the limbs. Usually, wine should be taken with hot water ; but when the progress of the case is satisfactory, alcohols are not necessary. All food should be taken hot, and prepared so as to please the taste of the patient.

EXERCISE AND EMPLOYMENT.

The patient should rise at 7 A. M., and take a walk for half an hour before breakfast at 8½ A. M. Exercise in the open air should also be enjoined for an hour or more before dinner, and again before tea. When engaged in business, half an hour or more must be employed at two periods of the day in exercise in the open air. He should retire to rest from 9 to 10 P. M. If there be much debility and sense of fatigue felt during the day, he should lie down on the couch before and after dinner, and particularly if he be tall, either absolutely or in relation to his age, and the action of the heart be feeble.

The exercise should be apportioned to the strength, but it should be carried as far as possible short of fatigue. When it can be tolerably borne it should be rough and free, as rapid walking, or moderate climbing, or running, or skipping, each of which is to be performed for limited periods at a time, and, if possible, with unvarying regularity as to the period of the day and duration. It should be made with a cheerful companion, and with as much *abandon* and gayety of feeling as possible. Men should walk, run, and climb, whilst women should walk briskly and skip, throwing the rope from before backwards, and resting when fatigued. Horse exercise is very proper for both sexes, unless there temporarily be much exhaustion. Riding in carriages is unworthy the name of exercise, except to those who are very feeble. Deep voluntary inspirations should be practised during ten minutes, twice a day, at the periods of exercise or otherwise.

The occupation should not be sedentary, nor be pursued in close or heated rooms, nor, in crowded places ; but out-of-door employment, under certain restrictions as to exertion and weather, is the most proper. A sitting occupation, in which the chest is leaning over a desk or the trunk is curved forward, is very injurious, and should be exchanged for the standing posture, but alternated at intervals with sitting. An occupation, also, which requires continuous standing should be avoided. Dust and irritating fumes are also injurious. The period of labour should be restricted to 6 P.M., and even to an earlier hour if it is practicable. But whilst there is commonly more to be feared than hoped for in the pursuance of the occupation of life by persons in this state of disease, it is, at the same time, of imperative necessity that the attention be moderately occupied through the day, and with an occupation which is felt to be profitable to the patient or to others, and within the sphere of his duty. Listlessness and idleness are particularly to be deprecated.

BATHING.

The patient should wipe the whole body over before retiring at night, and on rising in the morning, with a towel saturated with cold salt and water, and, in order to prevent the cold water trickling down the skin, the towel should be compressed a little before it is applied to the skin. The salt/ and water should be made with water which has been in the bed or other room during the day or night, and should be applied either immediately before or immediately after taking the cup of hot milk and chocolate. A dry, and perhaps rough, towel should be used afterwards with moderate freedom. Care should be taken to prevent much exposure, and particularly in cold weather, and the whole process should not occupy more than a minute or two. Men in tolerable health should use the plunge bath, or bathe in open water, for a few minutes every second morning. In the proper season, sea-bathing should be pursued every second day, but limited to three or five minutes.

CLOTHING.

The clothing should always be sufficient to maintain a comfortable warmth, without causing a sensation of heat or producing perspiration. Woollen vests and drawers should be worn by both sexes, but of different weights according to the season. They should not be worn during the night. Both the upper and lower extremities should be well clad, so as to prevent the sensation of cold, but if, notwithstanding the use of woollen clothing, they are cold, it is of the greatest importance to use rough friction and to apply external warmth, so as to induce the due amount of heat. The use of Indian-rubber goloshes is to be avoided, except whilst actually walking in the wet, and boots or shoes with cork and leather thick soles are to be preferred. We do not recommend patches of warm clothing with a view to render one part of the body hotter than another, and therefore rather deprecate the habit of loading the front of the chest with hare skins, chest protectors, or layers of flannel. The daily and general application of cold water will prevent local hyperæsthesia, and therefore the sense of necessity for this clothing; but, at the same time, the chest, both before and behind, must be kept comfortably warm by flannel shirts, high dresses, or double-breasted waistcoats. The neck should also be covered. The night covering should be moderate, and, if practicable, increased somewhat from 4 to 6 A.M. It should be quite sufficient to produce abundant warmth, but not perspiration or oppressive heat, and should consist of blankets, and not of *heavy* counterpanes. The face should not be covered by the bed-clothes, and there should not be any drawn bed-curtains.

The proper place for the bed is between the door and the window or fireplace, and not in a corner. If there should be too great a draught over the face, a curtain may be used to moderate its effect. The bed-room should be large and lofty, and, if possible, the patient alone, or, if married, the husband and wife should occupy the room. The bed-room should have the air moderately dry, and therefore it ought not to be on the basement or ground-floor. It should also be moderately cool, and, except when there is irritable cough, or the air damp, no fire should be lit in the room, and when a fire is used, charcoal should not be burnt, unless there is a good draught of air in the room.

RESIDENCE.

The house should be so well built that draughts from the windows and doors may be prevented. The roof should be sound and the ground floor made of wood, or, if of brick or stone, there should be wood placed upon it at the parts where it is used. No dampness of the floor or walls should be permitted.

A moderately dry, clear, bright, and cool atmosphere is the most fitted for this class of cases, and it must neither be very dry nor very moist. Westerly, northwesterly, or southwesterly winds are proper, and if they should blow strongly they are not be shunned. The north and the northeasterly winds are injurious and to be avoided, but they will be more tolerable when the temperature is moderately high with a north wind, and moderately low with an east wind. Rainy weather is undesirable, and the more so if it be very hot or very cold ; but in reference both to wind and weather, a moderately free exposure to them, when not extreme, is commendable. An extra covering should at all times be carried, when the patient is exposed to the weather, and whenever there is a sensation of cold, or when it varies, this should be employed, and no pains spared to regain the natural warmth as quickly as possible. A dry and frosty air is very salubrious, if the patient be not much troubled with cough, be able to take brisk exercise, and be sufficiently clad. When exposed to cool air, as on leaving the bed-room for the hall, or the house for the open air, the patient should close the mouth and breathe through the nose, and avoid speaking so long as the exposure continues. This is the effect produced when an artificial respirator is worn, and the closed mouth is the natural respirator.

The residence of the patient should not be low in relation to the surrounding country, nor in the immediate neighbourhood of a stream or lake. The ground should be well drained either by surface or sub-soil drainage, and in the summer time it may be either clay or gravel. There should not be any stagnant water in ditches or in irregularities of the ground, nor any source of fetid smells from decaying animal or vegetable matter. The house should be moderately elevated, but sheltered from the northeast. An open parklike country is to be preferred to a woodland district, and in the winter, or at very cold seasons, the town is to be preferred. The climate in the summer time should be northerly, and in the autumn the same, if the residence be near the deep sea or at the south, and in the winter southerly, or that of the healthy part of a very large town. There should be an absence of much rain and fog, or sudden changes of wind to the north.

MEDICINES.

In perhaps every case it is necessary to administer the mineral tonics : 15 minims of the tinct. ferri sesquichloridi, with or without an equal quantity of chloric ether, should be taken thrice a day in a wineglass of water, wine, beer, or quassia infusion ; or 8 grains of the citrate of iron and quinine thrice a day. The iodide of iron, when given, should be frequently intermitted. Cinchona and the mineral acids may be exchanged at intervals for the preparations of iron. Two or three drachms of cod-liver oil should be given twice or thrice a day, when it is tolerated. The condition of the menstrual function, the digestion and the alvine evacuation, will all need frequent attention. The best internal remedy for the cough is morphia in doses of 1-16 or 1-12 of a grain, taken every 4 or 6 hours with mucilage or syrup. Frequent examinations of the state of the pharynx should be made ; and this, with the state of the stomach and skin, will determine whether the acid or the alkaline plan of treatment must be temporarily pursued.

CHAPTER XXXVIII.

COD-LIVER OIL.

ALTHOUGH we have alluded to the action of cod-liver oil in other parts of this work, we think it necessary to discuss the merits of that substance in a yet more connected and minute manner. It is probable that no remedy for any disease has ever been more generally adopted than cod-liver oil in phthisis, not excepting, perhaps, quinine in ague. It is a remedy which was used at least so early as the time of Pliny, so far as regards some forms of disease, as rheumatism, gout, and scrofula, and its occasional employment was not forgotten by a few medical men in the 18th century; but as a remedy in phthisis, and in consideration of its universal use, it may be regarded as a new remedy, and one introduced to English practice so recently as 1841. It was most ably treated of by Dr. De Jongh in 1843, and again in his standard work entitled, "L'Huile de Foie de Morue, &c. Paris, 1853." To Dr. Hughes Bennett we owe, no doubt, its use in this country, since he first called attention to the great value which had already been attached to it on the continent of Europe.

We have said that within so short a period as twenty years its use has become universal over the whole civilized world, and we may well inquire as to the amount of good which it does afford, and the mode by which that good is effected.

It is quite true that new remedies have arisen from time to time, and, by that good or bad quality of the human mind by which so many act upon authority and are led by a leader, have gained celebrity and have been extensively used, but notwithstanding have been neglected and almost forgotten, a few years later; such, it may be inferred by the sceptical, may ere long be the fate of cod-liver oil. Yet we think that the universality of its use, both by confiding and sceptical minds, by the leaders and the led in the profession, places the merits of cod-liver oil on higher ground than that occupied by former favourites, and we cannot think that a remedy so approved can be otherwise than useful in the present condition of the human system. Hence we believe that it is a valuable agent, and one which is likely to remain in use, or lead to the introduction or general use of some other substance of an analogous nature. In the outset of our inquiry, then, we confess ourselves an advocate for its general use.

As the subject is one of so great interest and importance, we entered into an inquiry at the Hospital for Consumption, with a view to determine in what proportion of cases the use of cod-liver oil was beneficial, the direction of the relief which it afforded, and the relative advantage of its use when compared with that of other fats; and the results which were obtained are, we believe, substantially true.

In pursuing this inquiry, we sought for testimony in two directions, viz., both from the patient and the medical attendant. We questioned the 150 in-patients already referred to at page 48, as to their own opinion of the result and the mode of its action; and the following is the result of the inquiry, it being, however, understood that, in nearly every instance, other medicines were taken at the same time, and the separate influence of the oil could only be inferred.

85 stated that it benefited them; 16 stated that it benefited them at first, and injured them afterwards; 16 stated that it injured them; and 33 stated that it had no influence.

Thus those who were, in their own opinion, more or less benefited by it were 83 against 67, or 55 per cent. of the whole, or, if we add those on whom it was at first beneficial and afterwards injurious, 66 per cent. of the whole.

The mode in which they believed that it benefited them was variously stated. Thus, in their own words :—

Both stronger and stouter	.	22	Chest became stronger .	2
Stronger . . .	.	33	Less pain in the side . .	2
Stouter . .	.	13	Healed lungs . . .	2
Appetite improved .	.	8	Less pain in, or soothed, the	
Digestion " .	.	5	chest	6
Breathing " .	.	6	Less hoarse . . .	1
Cough " .	.	4	Did eyes good . . .	1
Chest " .	.	4	Nourished	2
Voice " .	.	1	Checked expectoration .	1
All respects . .	.	7	Prevented getting thin .	1
Removed sensation of sinking		1	Eased stomach . . .	1

In some instances the answers included two of the foregoing heads, and, although they were very dissimilar, it will be observed that in the great majority of the cases the benefit was referred to improved nutrition.

Of those who stated that they were not improved, or were injured, by the use of the oil,

36 were made sick.	1 had headache.
2 were made weaker.	2 found it never to agree.
6 had no appetite.	1 had been better since he
8 had oily eructations.	ceased to take it.
2 were made bilious.	

Thus, in nearly all this class of cases, the objections arose from the organs of primary digestion, as distinguished from the function of assimilation.

The cases comprehended all stages and conditions of the disease, and those who had taken the oil for periods varying from a few weeks to several years.

Such is the information as gathered from the statements of the patients; we will now question the medical report.

The medical report of these 136 cases, as furnished by the clinical clerks who watched the cases daily, showed that in 64 cases the disease was evidently progressing more or less quickly, in 43 it was apparently stationary, and in 18 there was an improvement. So that, in one half of the cases the disease advanced in spite of the cod-liver oil and other remedies, and in one-seventh there was apparent improvement of the lungs.

We then endeavoured to ascertain how far the amount of appetite for fat foot would correspond with the results from the administration of the oil, and the returns obtained prove the following :—

1st. In reference to the patients' report of the effects:

In 80 cases, in which benefit was received, three-fifths had appetite for all the fats, and one-fourth for three kinds, viz., butter, suet, and milk. In 29 cases in which the oil caused sickness or oily eructations, only 1 in 3½ had appetite for all fats, and 1 in 3 for butter, suet, and milk. It is also remarkable that, whilst in those who received benefit only 2 out of 80 had no appetite for fat and butter together, in those in whom the oil disagreed 11 in 29 had no appetite for fats.

Hence it follows that, where the oil was assimilated and was beneficial, there was much greater appetite for natural fats than where it was rejected in the first acts of digestion ; but it may not thence be inferred that wherever there is appetite for all fats in phthisis the oil would be beneficial, or *vice versâ*, for in 19 cases in whom no effect was produced, 10 could take all kinds of fat.

2d. The medical report showed that, of 43 in whom the disease was stationary, 28 could take all kinds of fat, and 8 could eat butter, suet, and milk ; and of 18 who were reported as improving, 10 could take all kinds of fat, and 7 could eat butter, suet, and milk. Hence from this report also we learn, that a majority of those who were improved during the use of the oil had appetite for the ordinary fats as food.

The facts elicited in this inquiry seem to be sufficiently definite, but we do not desire to attach too much importance to the precise percentage amounts, since it is probable that that would vary within certain limits in other similar inquiries ; but the general expression is in accordance with impressions derived from a consideration of many thousands of cases, and is, we believe, an approach to truth. This expression contains the following particulars :—

1. Cod-liver oil does not remove the disease.
2. The cases of permanent arrest of the disease are very few when compared with the whole.
3. Commonly the disease ultimately progresses, notwithstanding the use of the remedy.
4. In a large proportion of cases—about one-half—the progress is temporarily lessened.
5. The patient may report himself both stouter and stronger under the use of the oil, and yet the disease continue to advance.
6. When the oil disagrees with the patient, it is chiefly from its influence upon the digestive organs.
7. When its action is beneficial, it is chiefly by improving nutrition. Some remarkable instances of increase in weight have occurred under the combined influence of the oil, other remedies, the generous dietary of the hospital, rest and warmth ; and one of our out-patients gained 27 lbs. in weight. In an appreciable number of instances the patient is sensible of a local influence more or less apart from the general nutrition of the system. This local action is most important in the pharynx and other parts of the mucous tract to which the oil is directly applied.
8. There is a large class of cases in which it cannot be taken at all, and another in which, having been taken, it is not beneficial, and hence the use of it requires discrimination. As a rule, it is more commonly beneficial in those cases in which there is appetite for the ordinary fats in food, and it is commonly rejected when other fats are disliked, and hence the substitution of one kind of fat for another may be commonly effected.

MODE OF ACTION OF COD-LIVER OIL.

Having thus discussed the therapeutic value of this substance, we will proceed to consider its probable mode of action.

It has already been proved (page 48) that in a large proportion of phthisical patients there is a diminution of the quantity of fat which they take, and hence the natural presumption is that the oil meets this deficiency. The first point of interest is in reference to the cause of the lessened supply of fat in those patients who have the means of obtaining it. This is, we believe, due to one of two causes, viz., the lessened appetite for it, and the real or supposed evils which it induces. The latter is no doubt the rarer condition, since the ordinary answer to the inquiry is "I dislike it." This is also supported by the fact that if a patient dislike cod oil, he likes some other kind of fat; and by a judicious selection of fats, and a cautious and yet unflinching exhibition of them, the quantity taken may be greatly increased. It is contended that cod oil has special properties, which render its assimilation more easy than that of other fats, and hence among fats it is the most nutritive; but however true this may be in many cases, it is not by any means an universal truth. The inquiries just related show that in a large number of cases the oil is rejected by persons who can eat fat in food, and that even one-third of such persons take the fat of meat. If they can take fat in food, but not cod oil, it can scarcely show that the latter is more assimilable than the former. Moreover, in cases in which one kind of fat is objected to, the deficiency may be fully supplied by giving other kinds. Amongst the poor we find that many prefer pork fat, and affirm that it agrees better with them than any other fat. It must not be forgotten that mere dislikes are often very capricious and temporary, and as they arise, so may they pass away without reason; and this may be almost predicted if the judgment of a rational patient is appealed to, and that kind of fat be supplied which is the least distasteful. When the avoidance of fat really results from some imperfection in the digestive function, we believe that it always extends to cod-liver oil also, and it is matter of daily observation that in cases of disordered digestion cod-liver oil is not tolerated.

There are others who believe cod-liver oil to exert especial power by virtue of the amount of the hydrocarbons which it contains; but we do not see any ground for it except so far that, in comparing oils of somewhat different composition, care must be taken to administer as much of each kind as will afford the same elements.

The physical quality of viscidity is also one of great value, and in this cod oil and neats-foot oil stand pre-eminent. Where we desire to administer oil in the form of an emulsion, or to apply it locally to a mucous surface, and to have it retained upon the surface for as long a time as possible, as, for example, in throat affections, there can be no doubt that cod-liver oil has paramount claims to the attention. In this respect the dugong-oil is far inferior to cod-liver oil.

The received view of the mode of action of cod-liver oil is now clearer than was found at the general introduction of the oil into medical practice. At first, Dr. De Jongh, Dr. Bennett, and others attached value to the small quantity of iodine which it contains, viz., $\frac{3}{100}$ of a grain in each dose, and also to the phosphorus. Dr. De Jongh also believed that the various component elements of the oil had an action in their compound state much more beneficial than that which has been attributed to them when administered separately. In his work already quoted he writes at page 255: "Si nous considérons que dans les maladies où l'huile de foie de morue se montre d'une efficacité incontestable la digestion doit être relevée, la nutrition améliorée, les secrétions excitées, la fonction du système lymphatique vivifiée, et enfin—indication de la plus haute importance— que le système ganglionnaire doit être altéré; on se convaincra facilement que ni les principes de la bile, ni less matières grasses, ni l'iode, ni tout autre principe ne pourraient satisfaire chacun séparément à toutes ces indications. C'est pourquoi nous estimons devoir attribuer l'efficacité de l'huile de foie de morue, sinon à l'action combinée de tous ces principes, au moins à celle de la plupart d'entre eux." But whatever truth may be at the basis of this speculation, and particularly in reference to the scrofulous or tuberculous diathesis, we think that we shall be right in affirming that prolonged inquiry has led the profession to question these views in reference to phthisis in general, and to believe that to the fat must be attributed the good which is undoubtedly effected by this agent in the latter diseases.

Dr. Bennett affirms, on the theory of Dr. Ascherson, that the molecules of fat become coated with albumen, and constitute the molecules found in the chyle; and in this manner he asserts that cod-liver oil improves nutrition. This has been ably answered by Dr. Glover and Dr. Lawson, and the facts already cited in this book show that, whilst there may not be so much fat in the system in phthisis as is met with in health, there is never such a want as that a teaspoonful or a tablespoonful of oil could supply the defect, and it has not been proved that at all times there is not sufficient fat for the purpose referred to; moreover, it is well known that the increase of weight with the oil and food is oftentimes far greater than the improvement in nutrition could account for, and also that in numerous instances the tuberculization proceeds, notwithstanding the administration of the oil and the increase in the bulk of the body. Hence we think that whilst this theory may be a truth, it is far from being the whole truth.

In our experiments we have shown that fat always increases the fulness, and in some instances the rapidity of the pulse, and thus, in enfeebled conditions, will sustain capillary vital action. It also tends to lessen the action of the skin, and thus to prevent perspi-

ration and waste of heat; and we believe ourselves justified in asserting, that its action is to restrain elimination by every outlet of the
body, and thus to check loss of, and then to increase, weight.   It
is to this latter action principally that must be attributed the rapid
and great increase of weight which is frequently found to follow
the use of the cod-liver oil, and which is only temporary.

We fully agree with Dr. Bennett, Dr. Lawson, and most of the
writers of the day, as already stated, that the beneficial action of
cod-liver oil is due to its fatty quality, and we know that, as other
fats, it is liked by some and disliked by others, it is beneficial in
some and useless or even injurious in others; and often its place
may be advantageously supplied with any other fat which may be
preferred by the patient, provided it be taken in sufficient quantity
and with due regularity.   A prime reason of the good which has
resulted from the use of the cod oil is the regular supply of fat to
persons who otherwise would not have taken it in due quantity; and
a great merit in the introduction of it to general use is in having
led inquirers to prove the very important part which fat plays in the
animal system, and the real necessity for it which exists in all persons, and particularly in the young.

In concluding our observations, we may remark that it is of some
importance to determine the mode in which the oil may be the most
conveniently administered.   We have found much variety of taste
in the preference of the brown or pale oils; and whilst there are
many who prefer the pale, we believe that the mass of patients offer
no objection to the brown oil.   Moreover, considering the price,
the quality of the oil should be regarded, and yet it is well known
that other oils are commonly mixed with it.   We have been informed
by a manufacturer of cod-liver oil that probably not one-tenth of
the oil which is sold is altogether derived from the liver of the cod-
fish.   It is, however, impossible in private practice to determine
whether the oil which we prescribe is genuine cod-liver oil or not,
and hence we think it a great advantage that there is one kind of
cod-liver oil which is universally admitted to be genuine—the light
brown oil supplied by Dr. De Jongh.   It has long been our practice,
when prescribing the oil, to recommend this kind, since, amidst so
much variety and uncertainty, we have confidence in its genuineness.
As a rule we prefer that the patient should take it alone, since, by
so doing, the local effect is produced upon the fauces, and the dislike to it the sooner passes away.   It is also convenient to give it in
a wineglassful of hot milk, sweetened with loaf sugar, or with the
bitter infusions which are commonly prescribed with it, or in ginger
or orange wine, if such an adjunct be ordered; but where there is
an acid state of the secretions, or of the mucous membrane of the
throat, the stomach, or the duodenum, it is undoubtedly the best
plan to give it in the form of an emulsion with liquor potassæ, or to
administer an alkali with a bitter infusion a few minutes before the

oil is taken.   It is highly probable that an acid state of the intestinal tract is adverse to the due ingestion of the oil into the circulation.

CHAPTER XXXIX.

THE INFLUENCE OF CYCLICAL CONDITIONS.

In a work on the cyclical changes in the human system we have described in detail the variations in the vital functions which occur in the healthy system in the cycles of the day and the year, and we purpose here to apply the results thus obtained to the treatment of phthisis.

1. THE CYCLE OF THE DAY.

The chief points to be observed in the cycle of the day are the extreme variation between the day and night rate of the vital actions, the rapid and great increase which follows the meals, the equally rapid decrease which precedes them, and the lessened degree of action of food and similar agents in the evening.   These observations particularly apply to the rate of pulsation and respiration, and the quantity of air inspired and of carbonic acid expired.   In reference to the hourly elimination of urea, there is the greatest amount evolved at about mid-day, and this is followed by a great diminution until about 5 P.M., when, after tea, there is a second considerable increase until 8 or 9 P.M., and then the final fall of the night occurs. The hourly elimination of urinary water is the greatest after breakfast, and then a rapid decline occurs soon after mid-day.   There is but a small increase in the afternoon, and at length the quantity in the evening falls to that of the night, which is the least in the 24 hours.

But in phthisis it was found that all these hourly changes were exaggerated, so that the difference between the day and night rate was greater, and the variations due to food were greater, than in health.   The difference between the day and the night rate was an extreme of upwards of 40 pulsations per minute.   The rate of respiration was, in numerous cases, greatly increased in the early hours of the night with sleep; and indeed whenever sleep occurred by night or day, the rate of pulsation decreased, and that of respiration increased, during the continuation of the sleep.   This condition of the respiration is opposed to that in health, and was not universal in phthisical patients.   Hence, in reference to the treatment of phthisis, where the aim is to supply abundant nutriment and prevent failure of the vital powers, it is important that food be given in the night, to prevent too great a fall of the vital actions and the occurrence of profuse perspirations, and also in the early morning when the activity of the functions is great; and it is desirable that during the day the food be administered frequently, so as to avoid the great elevation and the subsequent great depression which occurs with ordinary meals at distant periods. Every care should also be taken at night, by means of warmth, clothing, &c., to prevent the great loss of temperature and to sustain the vital powers. Day sleep may be defended upon the same principle, for although there is at all times a depression of the vital actions with sleep, there is less with day sleep. It is also important not to administer much fluid in the early part of the day, lest the process of elimination should be unduly increased. We must refer further details to a paper published in the Medico-Chirurgical Transactions for 1856, which gives the result of an inquiry made at every hour during six days and nights without intermission, on three male and three female consumptives; but the general expression of the results is the importance of preventing too great a depression of the vital powers in the evening, during the night, and before meals, and too free elimination in the morning hours.

2. THE CYCLE OF THE SEASONS.

It is known that each season of the year has its own evil influences in cases of phthisis, so that with the heat of summer there is exhaustion, with the cold of winter inflammation, and at the changes of the seasons the liability to take cold, which either develops or increases the rapidity of the progress of the disease. As each of these conditions is explicable upon the principles recently eliminated by us in reference to the influences of season upon the animal system in health, and each requires careful consideration in the treatment of phthisis, we will now refer to the conditions of each season separately, but must refer to the work already quoted upon the cyclical changes for a more detailed statement.

In summer the rate of pulsation increases, whilst that of respiration declines. This was proved by us in an inquiry which we conducted on 15 in-patients during a whole month, in which we determined the rate of the two functions at 8 A.M. and 4 P.M. daily, and the results were published in Brit. and For. Med. Chi. Review for April, 1856. The quantity of carbonic acid and of air inspired decreases from the beginning of the hot weather in June to the end of August, and at the latter period the amount is only two-thirds of that at the former.[1] The skin is more active and sensitive. Hence in cases of early phthisis there is a rapid tendency to exhaustion of the vital powers as the summer advances, and this effect is particularly seen in July and August, after the long continuance of those conditions, so that there is less appetite for food, lessened powers of

[1] Phil. Trans., 1859.

assimilation, less innervation, less muscular power, and both shallower and feebler respiration—conditions precisely fitted to produce or to rapidly increase the disease. There is also profuse perspiration, inducing a soft and rapid pulse, with faintness from a deficient supply of blood to the head, and tendency to hæmoptysis from the rapid pulsation and increased tendency to congestion. Usually the cough abates, and the extremities remain warm, except after the profuse perspirations which occur in the early morning, when the skin, and even the breath, often feels cold. With the muscular relaxation which supervenes, the pupil dilates, and the power of locomotion is much reduced. In these conditions it is, therefore, highly important to avoid the sun's rays, to seek a cool and shaded room, to remain quiet, and even to doze during the middle hour of the day; to have food in a plain form, and often with some form of alcohol added (as two teaspoonfuls of brandy or rum to milk, or a small tumbler of hot and weak claret and water) every two hours, and also often in the night, and to use highly nitrogenized food; to vary the clothing carefully, both night and day, so as to lessen perspiration and prevent the cold which follows from it; to lessen the action of the skin by the external use of salt and water; to seek the seaside, or other suitable locality, where the circulation of the air is free and the temperature reduced.

On an examination of 177 cases of phthisis, we found that, when in good health, 51.4 per cent. bore heat badly, and 48.6 per cent. bore it well; so that the two classes were about equal in numbers. In cases of debility, the number of the former class was greater, viz., 71 per cent. This inquiry we deem of vital importance when we seek to estimate the probable influence of the hot season, or of change of residence to a warmer climate, and generally it will be found that as the system tolerates heat in health, so it will in phthisis.

In the winter the conditions of the system become more sthenic, and therefore in ordinary cases, and where the health is not materially reduced, and suitable protection given, this is a favourable season. We consider that a dry, cool air is the most beneficial in the cases in question. The evils of the season will, however, be the tendency to internal congestion and inflammation, the increase of cough from the irritation of the pharynx and air-passages, induced by the inhalation of cold air; the tendency to hæmoptysis from increased cough, irritability of the mucous membrane, and congestion of the lungs, and deficiency of temperature from the cold. If the patient be restricted to an artificially heated atmosphere, he will have the evils of dryness, stillness, and impurity of the air, and will be apt to have night perspirations from excess of clothing. Indeed, from whatever cause, night perspirations are common in winter. At this season the chief desideratum is the careful adjustment of the clothing, so that whilst the patient shall never be cold, he shall not be fatigued by the weight of many clothes; and the selection of an atmosphere so uniform and moderate in temperature, that he may be able to expose himself, at least under favourable circumstances. He should specially protect the throat, by keeping the mouth closed, and the throat externally covered, when in the open air. The clothing should be the best, and therefore the lightest, of woollen materials. The diet should be abundant, fat, and solid.

The change from the cold of winter to the warmth of early summer is attended by depression of the vital actions, and that in the autumn by the reverse, and the difficulty to be overcome is the inability of the system to adapt itself suddenly to the new conditions. Hence, with the fulness and high activity of spring, there is apt to be congestion of an active kind when the depressing influences of summer first act; and at the end of the year the tendency is to exhaustion, from the impossibility of the system to increase its vital changes with due rapidity. Hence disturbance of the circulation is common to both, but hemorrhage is more common in the spring; and internal congestions, with dropsical effusions, in the autumn. Moreover, it has always been observed that vascular congestions are found chiefly in the lungs in the spring, and in the chylopoietic viscera in the autumn. The indication in the spring is clearly to hold back the system, as by rest and the horizontal posture, and to avoid stimulants and excitants : whilst in the autumn the skin must be well protected, the vital powers sustained, and the patient altogether sheltered from the adverse conditions of the weather. It is well known to those who ride much on public conveyances that the horses get out of condition at the end of the year, and are unequal to their duties. Notwithstanding the occurrence of cold weather they perspire profusely, and need unusual protection and stimulating food.

It is needful to add a general remark in reference to the influence of season, that the effects are far more than the evident qualities of season—temperature, and weight of the air—can account for, as we have shown in the Phil. Trans., 1859, and also that an unusual state of the weather in any season induces conditions opposed to those ordinarily found at that season. Thus if, in winter, the temperature should be high, and the air moist, the patients immediately complain of all the conditions of body usually met with in the summer season, as exhaustion, defective appetite, feebleness, and perspirations. A temperature of 56° in mid-winter produces summer ill-effects, whilst the same at mid-summer would render the season winterly. It would appear that with the increase of the temperature from the winter, it is only as the sun increases in altitude and influence that the increase of heat is healthful to phthisical patients, and not simply the warmth which is due to the winds.

10

CHAPTER XL.

TREATMENT WITHIN HOSPITALS.

This subject is one of difficulty on account of its mixed character, for whilst the advantages and disadvantages offered by hospitals are almost fixed and determinate, the conditions required for the benefit of patients are very variable, and hence it would require a most extensive organization to meet the wants of even the great mass of cases.

The general hospitals have solved the problem by cutting, instead of untying the knot, and have rigidly excluded such cases, chiefly on the ground that they are irremediable, but also that the arrangements at such institutions are not favourable to the well-being of these cases. Hence special hospitals have arisen, into which the cases are received, but yet having arrangements almost identical with those of general hospitals.

It must be evident from the foregoing observations, that the class of cases under discussion cannot be efficiently treated in hospitals, unless those institutions have regulations and advantages specially adapted to them. Thus we have urgently recommended abundant and regulated exercise, a tolerably free exposure to the atmosphere, due amusement and occupation for the mind, abundance of milk for diet, and frequent and small meals, and, in addition, certain plans of ablution and voluntary respiration, which clearly demand the aid of others and the privacy of a separate bed-room. But how are these met even by the best arranged special and general hospitals? The patients are restricted to their rooms, or to long uninteresting corridors which have walls and high windows, or, if allowed to go outside, may saunter about paved yards or gravel walks, wet or dry, exposed to the gaze of passers-by, and with no shelter from the sun, wind, or rain. The space for out-of door exercise is very limited, and, from the nature of things, the exercise must be of such ordinary kinds as may not attract the attention of others. There is no gymnasium in which regulated muscular exertion may be made, and the mind be pleasantly engaged, nor any system adopted whereby the power of any special set of muscles may be increased. There is no plunging bath, warm or cold, in which the patients may seek tone, strength, and amusement. There are no games but such sedentary ones as draughts, and no bodily employment but such as making small woollen mats, by which a little money may be realized. There is no culture of the mind, except such as the clergyman may periodically offer and a small library afford, nor any such innocent pleasures as that of singing or instrumental music. The meals must be, as a rule, limited to three, or perhaps four, a day, at stated and distant periods, and it is impossible to supply to each patient the large quantity of milk which we have affirmed to be a prime necessity for the consumptive. Tea, sugar, and butter must be found by the patient, and hence be sparingly used whilst the action of the two latter is as important, probably, as that of cod oil conjoined with other articles of medicine. The amount of fat supplied in the dietary must be much less than that which the case demands, if the milk be limited to a small quantity, the meat not of the best-fed kind, and puddings containing fat be not commonly supplied, and hence they lack fat in food which should (but cannot) be given in oil. The temperature of the air is kept at an approach to uniformity, when it has been shown that the hourly variations occurring in the external air are conducive to health; and in the attempt to maintain it by artificial means, it often occurs that the temperature approaches 70° in the afternoon, and the degree of dryness of the air is increased to an extent which might be injurious. The windows and doors are sometimes doubled, so as to prevent ready access of the external air, and thus, with whatever care, the atmosphere within the hospital must be far less fresh and invigorating than that of green country fields. Indeed, the only conditions which are adopted are such as supply a tolerable amount of food, limit bodily and mental exertion, prevent the influence of low temperature, and afford medical treatment.

We affirm, therefore, unhesitatingly, that in the ordinary conditions met with in the early stage of phthisis, the arrangements of our hospitals are unsuited to the treatment of the case, provided the patient have a tolerable home in the country, with fresh air, green fields, and plain simple nutriment. They are, however, very valuable even at this stage in the exceptional cases in which there is an irritable cough, an inflammatory state of the throat, a tendency to inflammation of the lungs or to hæmoptysis, and in the winter season, and to all persons who have not a moderate amount of food and shelter. In practice it should be advised that such cases as have moderate shelter and food, and a country residence, should remain at home, whilst others may do well to gain admission.

Hence it follows that, in reference to this early or remediable stage of the disease, the necessary attention to the duties of life, and the greater advantages offered by the country, limit greatly the usefulness of such hospitals; and, indeed, they are chiefly suited to a more advanced condition, where there is hope of affording ease and comfort to the patient, and of somewhat prolonging his existence. Such institutions should, it is said, rather be termed homes or asylums than hospitals, since the benefit is derived as much from improved hygienic conditions as from medical treatment. But in order to this, the duration of the cases in the hospital should be lengthened much beyond the present narrow limits of two or three months, and thus avoid that relapse, and oftentimes more rapid progress, which occurs when the advantages of the hospital have ended, and the almost helpless patient is returned again to the privations of life.

Hence, on reflecting upon these questions, we are led in a degree to sympathize with the objections which are raised to the admission of such cases into general hospitals, where it is presumed that the prime object is the medical treatment, and where, consequently, cases of an acute nature are most fitly received. We would, however, very strongly support the effort which has recently been made to establish cottage hospitals in country localities, since, with intelligent administration, they might meet the wants of the mass of cases which we have been considering. We cannot doubt that every hospital, whether special or otherwise, receiving this class of cases, should have some cottage buildings suitably situated, to which the proper class of cases should be transferred, and thus reserve the hospital for those which are evidently more fitted for their present arrangements.

We have not included in these observations the attendance of out-patients at hospitals; for whilst we believe that to be the most interesting and valuable part of such institutions for the class of cases under consideration, the patients do not live within the walls.

CHAPTER XLI.

CLIMATE.

VOYAGING AND RESIDENCE.

THE indication offered by the disease in the selection of a suitable climate is to find the conditions in which tone of body may be improved without increasing the cough, or the tendency to inflammation of any part of the respiratory organs. This, we think, is a sufficient indication, and will enable us to point out those places which will be proper for the greatest number of patients, but it is evident that in each case we must estimate the relative importance of the two conditions according to the special liability to cough and inflammatory complications. It is also clear that as the seasons vary in character so must we seek different climates at the different periods of the year. We will first consider the cases fit for voyaging on the sea, and then the most suitable climates on land.

VOYAGING.

In the voyages to the East we have conditions which extend over three to four months in an unbroken chain, and if the voyage out and home be included a period of absence of nine to twelve months may be obtained. There is of course much diversity in the meteorological conditions met with in different latitudes, and in that sense the voyager to India or Australia may be said to pass through every temperate and torrid climate, but the mass of water and the motion of the water tend to maintain much more uniformity in conditions than occurs with so many climates on land. The air will vary in the amount of vapour which it contains, but it can never be a dry air, for an easterly wind passing over a large surface of water absorbs vapour, and is no longer dry. There is also every degree of movement of the air over the water, but commonly the movement is more uniform and of greater power than on land. There is also the greatest purity of the atmosphere. Hence in such a voyage there are the conditions of atmosphere which are suited to almost every case in the early stage of phthisis, viz., moderate temperature, tolerable uniformity in the hourly and daily temperature, moderate degree of moisture of the atmosphere, and a full average degree of motion of the air. The only modifying condition of the atmosphere unfavourable to our purpose is, that for a period of some weeks there will be exposure to the great power of the sun's rays, less, it is true, than is found in the same latitudes on land, and pleasantly counteracted by the sea breeze, but yet of higher temperature than we should desire. This is however to be obviated, to a great extent, by shelter and clothing, and is not sufficient to counterbalance the valuable qualities just mentioned, and much less so, when to these we add the avoidance of a multitude of evils inseparable from a residence on land and amongst masses of men. Moreover, the mode of life on shipboard may be rendered of the greatest service. Sea-sickness is an evil to which nearly all persons are liable, but commonly it passes away within forty-eight hours, and after the lapse of a few days it is almost or quite forgotten. There is an utter absence of daily care, and a delightful sense of freedom is obtained within a few days of this exclusion from general society. The contemplative who love retirement, and the merry who rejoice in jollity and good humour, find in the quiet and regularity of a life upon the sea, and the companionship of sailors, that which meets their wants. It is to this, we believe, that must be attributed the indescribable charm which the sea offers to the real sailor, and is identical with the deep sense of security and freedom which takes possession of the heart of the trapper who, in the distant solitudes of the far West, will have no companion but his horse and dog—a state of feeling, however, *toto cœlo* removed from that of the misanthropist. To these we must add the simple, abundant, and regular meals which are supplied in all well-regulated ships, and the invitation which is ever present to spend the hours of the day in the open air.

There are, however, two circumstances which call for arrangement, viz., the occupation and the sleeping room. It is of great importance that the voyager have a daily occupation, either in the affairs of the ship, or one entered into for his own gratification, so that his attention may be healthfully employed. Hence we recommend such patients as may be able to obtain a nominal engagement on shipboard, taking care as to its duties and the food which will be supplied; but as this is not always attainable, it is better for them to lend a hand at the ropes, and to practise mounting the yards, to engage in the games played upon deck, or to have some scientific investigation in hand. In reference to the sleeping-room, it is certainly of prime importance that it should be sufficiently large and ventilated, and be free from the foul odor of bilge water, or other decomposing matters, and the offensive smells of the engine-room. A sleeping berth upon the deck is much better than one below.

Voyaging in the South Pacific Ocean has the further advantage of offering even greater uniformity of climate, and of presenting scenes with which the European mind is not familiar, and is a very valuable agent for the purpose now under discussion.

The voyage to the Northern States of America is now reduced to so short a period that it loses much of its advantages for our purpose; for if it be made in a sailing-vessel, it will almost always be performed within three weeks, and if the object be to remain upon the sea for a period of many months, there will be the great disadvantage of perpetual change of climate, and of frequent delays in port. Moreover, in proceeding to the New England States or to Canada, there is the disadvantage of the cold experienced on approaching New Foundland, with its fleet of partially dissolved icebergs, unless the course be directed more southerly so as to reach the Gulf Stream. In a sailing-vessel it frequently happens that the proximity to New Foundland influences the temperature of the air for a week, and causes both a sudden and a prolonged effect upon the system.

In reference to the period of the year when the voyage may be most suitably undertaken, we may remark that to America it must be in the summer season, viz., from May or June to September, but to the East it matters but little at what period of the year it is undertaken. It is, however, better to leave England in the spring, so as to reach Australia in the winter season, or any period from November to August.

It is not necessary to enter upon any attempt to select the fitting cases for voyaging, since, so far as the disease is concerned, all at the stage in question are suited, and the selection of this or other plans of treatment will depend less upon the condition of the patient than upon other and non-medical considerations. We think it should be carried out for a period of not less than one year, and if possible it should extend over two years. The patient should be suitably provided with the varieties of clothing required, and with the exception of some details in diet, as, for example, the comparative absence of milk, he will be able to pursue the whole plan of treatment.

The voyage to America is less fitted for those who suffer from irritability of the pharynx and larynx, and in whom changes of temperature produce cough and dyspnœa, than for those in whom atony seems to be the characteristic feature. The former class should certainly proceed to the East or to the Southern Seas, whilst the latter may take either at pleasure.

RESIDENCE ON LAND.

In reference to the indications already mentioned, we think that the following conditions should be sought for in selecting a suitable place of residence.

1. As cool a temperature as is compatible with the prevention of irritation of the air passages.

2. The least daily variation of temperature.

3. The least hourly variation of temperature.

4. Moderate amount of moisture in the air, and therefore little or no fog.

5. Moderate movement of the atmosphere.

6. General absence of northeast or easterly winds in this climate, and hot dry winds abroad.

7. The air free from foul odours and smoke.

8. All the conditions as to society, scenery, and food which are the most conducive to bodily health and mental enjoyment.

The year may be practically divided into the winter and summer half-years, April or May, and October or November being the dividing months; for although the spring and autumn are periods of great anxiety in the cases now under discussion, it will be safer to add them to the summer and winter periods respectively.

In discussing the meteorological conditions of the summer and winter residences, we shall select from the Registrar-General's returns those of the six years which approach the present period, viz., from 1855 to 1860, both inclusive. We shall include those of six months, July to December, in the summer, and those of three months, January to March, in the winter resorts.

The subjects of inquiry will be the mean temperature, the mean daily range, the extremes of temperature, the degree of saturation of the air, and the prevalent direction of the winds. It will also be borne in mind that we shall refer only to those conditions which are suited to cases of phthisis in the early stage.

CHAPTER XLII.

CLIMATE.

SUMMER CLIMATES.

WE will now consider the climates which are suitable for the summer and autumnal periods, or for parts of these periods respectively, but in doing so we must remark *in limine* that our object is not to write a treatise upon climate, but only to point out the leading advantages of the localities, which we recommend in the treatment of the disease, and the stage of disease, in question.

As a general expression we state that during the summer half-year the conditions above mentioned can be found only in certain positions at the sea-side. In all inland districts the effect of variations of temperature is great, and is immediately felt, so that there is much hourly variation between the day and the night, and much variation from day to day. Moreover, as the summer advances the ground absorbs heat, and the effects of high temperature are thus continued after the highest temperature of the air has passed over. Hence the general effect of temperature is considerable, and increases by duration, and it lessens all the vital changes.

At the sea-side, on the contrary, in situations where there is great depth of water up to the shore, the temperature is much less than in inland districts, and is more uniform both hourly and daily. The reason of this is clear, since the temperature of the sea-water in summer is much lower than that of the air and soil, and consequently the greater the proportion of sea-water and the more the air passes over it the lower will be the temperature of the locality in the summer. We must, therefore, seek not only for the sea-side, but for great depth of water up to the coast, and if possible, in addition, a position where the prevailing wind blows over the sea. The temperature must, however, remain so high that the cooler winds shall not so lower it that the vapours must be precipitated and fogs be produced. We will now refer to a few localities which appear to us to meet most of these requirements.

SCARBOROUGH.

We take it for granted that, with the conditions already laid down, we must select some northern sea coast during the summer half-year, and in doing so our first choice must be the queen of northern watering places.

This favourite place is an ancient fishing town, built on the very margin of a fine bay, at a point where the bank shelves down somewhat abruptly to the beach, having on either hand a large range of high and precipitous cliffs. Hence there is a hollow central part, and two elevated wings. the former constituting the old town, and the latter the south and north cliffs; and in addition there is a remarkable projection of rock extending far out to the sea, at the end of the north cliff, affording a tolerably large plateau, upon which are the ruins of the ancient castle. The bay is open to the north and east, and whilst the north cliff is fully exposed to both these winds, the central part of the town is sheltered from the north by the large mass of the castle rock. The south cliff is fully exposed to the east and southeast, but there are parts in an intervening valley where the houses have a southerly aspect. The elevation of the tide in the harbour is moderate, and whilst the recess of the tide is sufficient to allow of a handsome promenade at low water, the high tide reaches the cliff, except at the part of the coast where the town is built. Hence the depth of water is very considerable, and it is even at low water close upon the town.

The mean temperature of the air during each month of the summer and autumn quarters was as follows in the six years 1855 to 1860 :—

TABLE No. 11.

Mean Temperature.

	1855	1856	1857	1858	1859	1860
	°	°	°	°	°	°
July	56.8	57.3	59.6	56.7	60.2	54.1
August	59.3	57.6	59.7	58.3	60.2	54.6
September	54.7	52.6	57.3	56.6	54.2	50.8
Means	56.9	55.8	58.8	57.2	58.2	53.2
" Greenwich . . .	60.4	59.9	63.3	61.	62.7	56.2
October	48.3	50.8	52.3	49.2	47.9	48.6
November	43.9	42.	46.8	42.8	41.8	42.4
December	37.5	40.9	45.	40.2	35.9	36.7
Means	43.2	44.6	48.	38.9	41.8	42.2
" Greenwich . . .	42.7	44.2	47.9	43.8	43.2	42.2

The average temperature of each of the two quarters was thus 56.7° and 43.1°, whilst that of a favourable inland place, the Royal Observatory at Greenwich, was 60.6° and 44.3°. Hence the average temperature at Scarborough was, as compared with that at Greenwich, lower in both summer and autumn.

The extremes of temperature, and the range between the highest
and lowest temperature, in each month, were as follows :—

TABLE No. 12.

Extremes of Temperature.

		1855	1856	1857	1858	1859	1860
		°	°	°	°	°	°
July	Highest	75.5	74 5	66.9	72.	77.4	69.7
	Lowest	48.	42.3	54.9	46.2	53.5	40.
August . . .	Highest	74.	75.1	65.5	71.6	74.5	64.
	Lowest	50.3	48.3	57.	46.3	49.	46.5
September .	Highest	69.5	61 3	61.8	67.5	66 2	61.
	Lowest	45.	41.	54 5	46.	45.	40.
October . . .	Highest	59.5	53.3	61.5	62.	64.5	58.
	Lowest	35.	48 4	39.	38.	27.	33.
November . .	Highest	51.5	44.9	55.8	51.	50.5	59.
	Lowest	33.4	37.8	31.	29.	32.5	28.
December . .	Highest	47.6	44.	58.	52.2	50.	46.
	Lowest	22.2	36.8	32.	30.	14.5	16.

The extremes of temperature in the summer quarter were 77.4°
and 40° ; and in the autumn quarter 64.6° and 16°. The extreme
difference of temperature was thus 37.4° in the summer, and 48.5°
in the autumn ; but it is evident that the latter is beyond the ordinary extremes, since the lowest temperature of that year was much
below the lowest temperature of other years.

The mean daily range of temperature at the same periods was as
follows :—

TABLE No. 13.

Daily Range of Temperature.

	1855	1856	1857	1858	1859	1860
	°	°	°	°	°	°
July	9 4	13.3	12.	10.7	5.4	8 5
August.	10.7	7.9	8.5	9.6	10.5	8.4
September . . .	9.2	7.9	7.8	8.2	8.8	6.9
Means	9.8	9 7	9.2	9.5	8.3	7.9
" Greenwich . . .	19.7	20.	21.	21.2	21.5	17.4
October	6.5	4.9	6.2	6.8	6.5	6.9
November	4.6	7.1	4.9	5.	6.4	4.6
December	6.1	7.2	6.6	5.7	7 3	4.
Means	5.7	6.4	5.9	10.3	6.7	5.1
" Greenwich . . .	10.8	11.7	12.2	12.4	12.5	11.3

The average daily range of temperature was, therefore, so small
as 9.0° and 6.6°, whilst that at Greenwich was 20.1° and 11.8°, or
an amount more than double of the range at Scarborough.

The amount of moisture in the atmosphere in relation to the production of fog may be most conveniently ascertained by determining the degree of approach to saturation of the air, for when the air is saturated, at whatever temperature, any further attempt at increase of vapour, or any diminution of the temperature, must cause a deposition of vapour. Complete saturation is represented by 100, and the approach to it will be indicated by the number below that amount, as in the following table.

TABLE No. 14.

Degree of Saturation of the Air.

	1855	1856	1857	1858	1859	1860
July	91	82	84	87	80	92
August	87	87	91	89	93	83
September	83	83	88	92	97	86
Means	87	84	87	89	86	87
" Greenwich . . .	79	77	77	73	72	84
October	90	85	89	92	90	80
November	90	85	92	94	98	91
December	88	87	92	94	96	90
Means	89	86	91	91	94	87
" Greenwich . . .	87	89	92	87	88	91

The average approach to saturation was thus 86 and 88 as compared with 100, whilst that at Greenwich was at the same periods 77 and 89. Hence it follows that whilst the air was not saturated it contained a considerable amount of moisture in relation to its temperature—an amount relatively greater than that at Greenwich in the summer, but not greater than that at Greenwich in the autumn quarter. It is far removed from being a dry air, and is not an extremely moist air.

The prevalent direction of the wind in the months in question preponderates greatly in one quarter, as is proved by the following figures, which show the relative frequency of the wind from each quarter of the compass. In 1855 the general direction is alone given in the returns :—

Prevalence of Winds.

	July.				August.				September.			
	N.	E.	S.	W.	N.	E.	S.	W.	N.	E.	S.	W.
1855	S. W.				N. W. & S. E.				S. W. & N E.			
1856 . .	8	5	22	27	13	14	18	17	11	14	15	.19
1857 . .	4	3	9	15	13	6	8	9	8	7	9	7
1858 . .	7	6	8	10	9	7	9	6	8	8	12	12
1859 . .	4	3	5	4	2	3	3	4	5	...	9	14
1860 . .	12	11	4	4	11	7	5	8	9	6	7	8

	October.				November.				December.			
	N.	E.	S.	W.	N.	E.	S.	W.	N.	E.	S.	W.
1855	S. W. & W.				Variable.				N. W. & S. W.			
1856 . .	4	10	25	23	19	2	10	29	19	3	6	34
1857 . .	6	8	9	8	7	7	6	10	1	1	10	19
1858 . .	9	5	4	13	6	8	6	10	5	1	11	16
1859 . .	4	8	6	5	5	6	11	8	3	3	12	11
1860 . .	6	3	10	12	5	17	8	5	5	14	12	2

Thus on the average of each quarter the relative number of east winds was 17.6 and 18.2, and that of the west was 32.8 and 42, showing a vast preponderance of westerly winds, and when the northern and easterly, and the south and westerly are respectively added together, it will be seen that the relative numbers of the former are 41.5 and 39 against 60.4 and 69.2 of the latter. The west wind is two and a half times as prevalent as the east wind, and the south are one-quarter more prevalent than the north, whilst the southwest winds are more than one-half more prevalent than the northeast winds. Hence at Scarborough there is, during the periods in question, a manifest prevalence of the west and southwest winds ; and as the aspect of the sea is north and east, it follows that the wind is for the most part a land wind, and does not therefore exert the influence over the temperature of the place which would occur if it were a sea wind. The difference of temperature on a bright summer's day between the air at the top of the cliffs and that on a level with the water is very considerable, so that the latter is the most desirable place at that period.

The occurrence of fog is comparatively rare, since the temperature is never very high in the summer nor very low in the autumn, and as the former restricts the capacity for the reception of vapor, and the latter does not greatly lessen it, it follows that the air does not readily become saturated with moisture and precipitate the excess in the form of fog. When fog occurs it is for the most part due to the injection of a northeasterly wind, which, whilst traversing a portion of the bay from north to south, precipitates the vapor in the lower region of the air, and even in that which covers the cliffs, but it does not occur at an elevation at a short distance from Scarborough.

Hence we have shown that there are nearly all the conditions required in the treatment of early phthisis found at Scarborough in the summer and autumn months, viz., low summer and high autumn temperature, with small daily range and a moderate amount of moisture, and we may further state that they often extend into January, and in our judgment it is a locality well fitted for the reception of this important class of cases. There is also the great advantage of a beautiful marine promenade, of a fine hilly surrounding neighbourhood, and of numerous excursions, both by land and water, during the season.

The south cliff is said to be warmer than the north cliff, and whilst this is true, it may be well to state that at present the inhabitants underrate the value of the north cliff. The south cliff has no doubt the merit of being gay and fashionable, of being near to the spa, and of enjoying a beautiful view of the town and bay, but on the north cliff there are the great advantages of a cooler and more bracing air in the summer months, a fine clear sea, proximity to the castle rock, and above all, so much quietude that, as the view of Scarborough is shut out from it, it has the advantage of being itself a small watering place.

The town has for several generations been a watering place of note, but it has increased most rapidly within the last fifteen years, so that nearly the whole of the fine ranges of houses on the north cliff, and a large part also of the south cliff, have been built within that period. It is abundantly supplied with accommodation for visitors, particularly of the middle and higher classes, and offers some sheltered spots for invalids. The castle rock is a most picturesque object, and the crown of it a most elevated and healthful promenade, and if the inhabitants were somewhat more fond of the beautiful, they might make walks upon its side overlooking the town, and by this rock, and a marine promenade to be built from its foot along the shore to the south cliff, make this the most magnificent resort in the kingdom.

There are also other places upon the same coast which offer similar advantages to the class of patients under consideration, as for example, Filey, Burlington, and Whitby. Filey is suited to those who seek quietude, and Whitby has the advantage of a beautiful neighbourhood, with pleasant walks and drives, but whilst they each have special advantages and are well fitted for the temporary residence of cases of early phthisis, we think them by no means equal to Scarborough for the purpose in hand.

THE ISLE OF MAN.

We have placed the Isle of Man second upon our list on account
of its distance from the greater part of England, the necessary journey across the channel, the shorter period during which patients
may remain there, and the comparatively limited accommodation which
it affords, but in truth, in reference to its fitness in a medical aspect,
as a short and temporary residence for cases of early phthisis, we
believe it to be scarcely rivalled ; and moreover, those who are acquainted with the stormy periods of its history and its unique social
and political institutions, will find much material for study and amusement, whilst they at the same time gain the treasure for which they
visited its shores.

It is, as is well known, a small island about twelve miles in
breadth and thirty-four miles in length, and consequently, whatever may be the direction of the wind, a sea breeze must float
over the whole of it. It is surrounded by deep water on every
shore, so that it has on all sides the means of maintaining an approach to uniformity of temperature, and in the summer period as
the prevailing winds must come over the sea, they reduce the temperature of the air in the inland districts. The shores are precipitous on all sides except at the northern part of the island, and the
water which washes them is of the clearest blue colour. In the
interior of the island there are ranges of mountains running northeast and southwest, and in the north-central part of the island these
form a basin of moderate dimensions. The height of the highest
mountain, Snaefield, is 2200 feet, and that of the range varies from
900 to 1500 feet. There are also numerous narrow dells and valleys in which are torrent-like streams, which afford good sport for
the angler. On the tops of the hills the pure sea breeze is constantly felt, and in the chain extending in the north-central direction, it is possible to travel leisurely for several days without
descending into the valleys, except for the night. Moreover, the
cliffs which rise up from the shores are elevated and well exposed to
the breeze, and particularly on the southern and western sides of
the island, afford unlimited opportunities for the most healthful
exertion. Hence from the surrounding deep water, the perpetual
sea breeze, the high cliffs and the comparatively large ranges of
low mountains, with rounded summits, the island is particularly
adapted to give tone to those who seek it, whilst the valleys being
numerous, deep and narrow, offer shelter and a warm and moist air
in the hot season.

The chief towns are five, viz., Douglas, Peel, Castletown, Ramsay, and Laxey, the first and two last situate on the east, and the
second on the west shore, whilst Castletown, the seat of the Government, is on the south, and away from the sea. There are
numerous farm dwellings and some villages in the inland districts,
but they are not such, for the most part, as could be occupied by

visitors, and it is to be regretted that there are no habitations built upon the elevated sides of the mountain ranges. Hence the visitor is compelled to reside in one of the towns named, and of these undoubtedly Douglas, with its magnificent bay, is the most frequented; and with Peel, on the western shore, is the most beautifully situated. But when wandering for days together over the summits of the hills inhaling the dry, cool, sea-breeze, with its invigorating and inspiriting influences, and here and there lying down amongst the heather and gathering the scattered bilberries, the visitor may probably long to live in tents for a season, or wish that houses were built, which would render it unnecessary to descend behind the hills, which cut off the sea breeze, and traverse valleys where the warmth, moisture, and stillness of the air impede respiration, and relax the system.

In these mountain ranges, once covered with fir trees, but now quite bare, the island possesses wealth which it has neither appreciated nor realized; and as, owing to the peculiar tenure of the land, and the jealousy of the inhabitants in asserting their rights against Imperial claims, it is yet impossible that the land can be used for other purposes than those of the common right. We venture to predict that when the value of that locality as a restorer of health shall be acknowledged, and residences be provided, it will become a summer resort of the greatest value to the middle classes of England.

We are enabled by the aid of the Quarterly Returns of the Registrar General to show the meteorological conditions which belong to the island, and we will analyze them in the manner already related in reference to Scarborough, selecting the years 1855 to 1860 inclusive.

The following table shows the mean monthly temperature of the air:—

TABLE No. 16.

Mean Temperature.

	1855	1856	1857	1858	1859	1860
	°	°	°	°	°	°
July	58.8	55.	57.1	56.1	60.2	56.2
August	57.1	59.6	60.2	58.	57.9	54.8
September	54.1	53.3	56.5	56.5	53.7	...
Means	56.7	56.	57.9	56.9	57.2	...
" Greenwich . . .	60.4	59.9	63.3	61.	62.7	...
October	49.	52.4	52.7	49.1	50.2	49.5
November	48.2	44.7	47.	43.1	44.4	42.9
December	39.5	42.4	48.9	44.7	38.	38.2
Means	43.9	46.5	49.5	45.6	44.2	43.5
" Greenwich . . .	42.7	44.2	47.9	43.8	43.2	42.2

The temperature was thus on the average of five years in the summer and autumn quarters 56.9° and 45.9°, and whilst slightly lower than that of Scarborough in the summer, it was higher in the autumn of the same years.

TABLE No. 17.

Extremes of Temperature.

			1855	1856	1857	1858	1859	1860
July	. . .	Highest	77.4	72.	73.7	71.7	74.9	75.
		Lowest	42.7	39.	43.5	44.7	45.6	43.4
August . .	.	Highest	73.9	82.1	81.	79.1	74.	69.
		Lowest	42.1	42.6	46.2	43.6	45.	40.
September	.	Highest	69.5	68.8	73.	73.4	68.1	...
		Lowest	58.	39.8	41.2	40.8	38.	...
October .	.	Highest	66.9	65.	64.8	64.4	66.3	63.7
		Lowest	31.	43.5	36.9	32.9	29.6	31.9
November	.	Highest	54.8	58.1	57.8	56.1	56.1	56.
		Lowest	28.9	27.6	25.9	27.8	29.5	29.4
December	.	Highest	49.9	57.1	56.5	54.	52.9	49.1
		Lowest	24.3	22.	32.	31.5	10.3	12.

The daily range of temperature was as follows:—

TABLE No. 18.

Range of Temperature.

	1855	1856	1857	1858	1859	1860
July	17.2	16.3	16.8	16.9	16.5	16.2
August	14.5	15.7	16.7	18.3	17.4	14.3
September	15.3	13.7	15.3	14.1	16.	...
Means	15.7	15.2	16.8	16.4	20.	...
" Greenwich . . .	19.7	20.	21.	21.2	21.5	...
October	14.2	8.7	10.4	11.8	12.5	10.4
November	10.1	9.5	10.	10.4	10.5	7.5
December	8.8	9.4	7.2	7.7	11.2	8.3
Means	11.	9.2	9.2	10.	11.3	8.7
" Greenwich . . .	10.8	11.7	12.2	12.4	12.5	11.3

The average daily range of temperature during the two seasons was somewhat considerable in the summer quarter, and amounted to 16.6° and 9.9° at the two seasons. The average was considerably higher than that of Scarborough, but much lower than that at Greenwich. It is no doubt due to the influence of the mountain range over the temperature of the lowland parts where the observations were made.

The degree of saturation of the air with vapour is thus represented, the full saturation being regarded as 100.

TABLE No. 19.

Saturation of the Air.

	1855	1856	1857	1858	1859	1860
July	91	88	93	88	89	92
August.	91	82	86	88	87	97
September	86	84	91	91	84	...
Means	89	86	90	89	86	...
" Greenwich	79	77	77	73	72	...
October	85	87	90	87	90	88
November	82	83	90	85	89	89
December	84	88	90	93	92	92
Means	84	86	90	88	90	89
" Greenwich	87	89	92	87	88	91

Thus the average degree in two seasons was 88 and 87.8, which was a little higher in the summer and a little lower in the autumn than at Scarborough, and therefore was higher in the summer and lower in the autumn than at Greenwich.

The prevailing direction of the wind in the various months was as follows :—

TABLE No. 20.

Prevalence of the Winds.

	July.				August.				September.			
	N.	E.	S.	W.	N.	E.	S.	W.	N.	E.	S.	W.
1855		W.			S. W. & N. W.				——			
1856 . .	8	3	9	21								
1857 . .	4	0	9	18	9	7	8	7	5	6	12	7
1858 . .	6	4	7	14	9	3	9	10	3	6	10	11
1859 . .	2	6	7	12	2	2	12	11	11	7	3	9
1860 . .	9	3	5	7	9	4	6	11				

	October.				November.				December.			
	N.	E.	S.	W.	N.	E.	S.	W.	N.	E.	S.	W.
1855		W.			N. & N. E.				Variable.			
1856 . .					17	5	4	8	19	4	15	23
1857 . .	4	8	9	10	6	13	7	4	3	1	12	15
1858 . .	6	6	6	13	8	14	5	3	3	2	14	12
1859 . .	4	3	6	5	5	6	11	8	3	3	12	11
1860 . .	6	6	5	14	6	6	10	8	12	10	7	2

The observations are unfortunately incomplete, but by a suitable calculation it may be seen that the relative number in the two quarters was, east 12 and 18, west 34 and 29, and when the north-east and the southwest are respectively considered together, the former are 31 and 40 against 58 and 55. Hence the westerly and southwesterly winds greatly prevail over the easterly and north-easterly, and the larger proportion of the latter occurs in the autumn quarter.

On a review of these results it will be observed that there is a substantial agreement between the meteorological condition of Scarborough and the Isle of Man, except that the daily range of temperature and the variability of the wind are greater at the latter than at the former.

Our friend, Mr. Oswald (the oldest medical man in the Island, we believe, and formerly the medical attendant of the recent Lord of the Island, the Duke of Athol), has given much attention to this subject, and with great intelligence has accumulated a mass of facts through fifty years of much interest, in their relation to disease. It is deeply to be regretted that the scientific world has not hitherto been favoured with the results of his labours.

But it must be evident that observations made in the interior and lowlands of the Island will vary very much from any which might be made on the mountain ranges, and it is to be regretted also, that no precise information has hitherto been obtained from the latter. It is well understood that in the winter season the force of the wind is very considerable, and that the northerly winds which then prevail, cause great coldness on the mountains, and also that, as in all mountainous districts, drizzling rains are apt to occur in all seasons; but for the summer months of June, July, August, and September, we fearlessly recommend this as one of the best resorts for the cases under consideration, in whom there is no marked tendency to inflammatory action. Until recent years the class of visitors to the island was very select, and the numbers were few, but now the numbers are great—greater indeed than Douglas is fitted to accommodate, and consist largely of the working classes.

There is abundant accommodation for visiting the various parts of the island, and the pedestrian will find from the Calf of Man to Ramsay sufficient opportunities for climbing; whilst from its high cliffs he may watch a fleet of from 100 to 200 vessels engaged in fishing, and beyond it the mountains of Scotland to the west, and those of Cumberland to the east. There are also opportunities of proceeding to Whitehaven for the Lakes and to Scottish shores. Whilst, therefore, there is much of the country which looks inhospitable, the inhabitants poor, and the institutions belong to an earlier era, the patient will yet find much to interest him in the natural scenery—something to admire in the hospitable feeling of the people, and temptation to seek health and vigour in the remarkably elastic and bracing atmosphere of the hill ranges.

THE ENGLISH LAKE DISTRICT.

The district of the Cumberland and Westmoreland lakes is so extensive, and offers so great a variety of conditions, that it may seem valueless to refer to it as a whole, and yet for the purposes of this work we think that minute detail is unnecessary. The general impression which we entertain is that this district is not suited to the classes of cases now under consideration as a residence for any considerable period. In the diversity of scenery which exists, and which offers so great charms to the pedestrian, it must be borne in mind that the only places in which a patient may reside are the valleys, and the neighbourhoods of the lakes and streams ; and in most of these parts the summer heat with the moisture renders the atmosphere oppressive and relaxing. There are none of the mountains which are adapted for habitations ; so that whilst the mountain air is most desirable, it can only be obtained by much exertion, and its good effect is counteracted by the conditions of the valleys.

In these remarks, however, we have in view the cases in which the sole object is to give tone to the system, and where there is not the desire or ability to spend the whole period in travelling ; but in the cases in which there is a tendency to inflammatory action, or to much irritability of the air-passages, there are many parts of these districts which are well suited to them. Such are for example, the higher shores of Windermere, or the head of Grasmere Lake, and, above all, the charming neighbourhood of Keswick. These cases are, however, comparatively few, and it would require great care to prevent the peculiar conditions of the valleys from lowering the tone of the system.

Upon the whole we do not regard the English lakes as well suited for the residence of the class of cases under consideration.

SCOTLAND.

The class of cases to which a summer residence in Scotland is well fitted, is such as are able to make a considerable amount of exertion, either on foot or horseback, and who find special enjoyment in mountain scenery and in sauntering among the heather. To those of less bodily vigour, and especially to all such as suffer from irritable cough, much better summer residences may be found.

The parts of Scotland which are the most suited to our purposes are : 1st. The routes usually taken by tourists, where the desire of the patient is rather to travel than reside, and of these, none excel that from Glasgow to Inverness ; or 2d, the beautiful neighbourhoods of Dunkeld and Blair Athol, or those of Ballater and Braemar, where every facility is met with both for residence and travel ; and 3d, an island situation as that of Skye.

There is one general observation which applies to all these regions with considerable force, viz., that there are extremes in the daily range of the thermometer, so that, with the nights cool or cold, the influence of the midday sun is very considerable; also, that the air is for the most part so near to saturation, and that the injection of a cooler wind causes a deposition of vapour, and the well-known Scotch mists are produced. Hence, as a residence, they can never be well suited for the class of cases under consideration; but in fine seasons, or for such part of the season as the weather may remain fine, and for travelling and residing alternately for limited periods, they offer many advantages. Upon the whole, we commend the selection of the Isle of Skye, or of some other of the northern islands; but there, as in other parts of the Highlands of Scotland, there is difficulty in obtaining a ready supply of fresh meat and other necessary food suited to the invalid traveller.

The most suitable period of the year is from the middle of June to the middle or end of August.

NORWAY.

The remarks which we have made in reference to Scotland apply, in a great degree, to Norway; but the latter is more exclusively a place for the traveller than for the resident. Its deep fiords on the one hand, and pine forests on the other, tend much to equalize the temperature—the former modifying the summer heat, and the latter the autumn cold. It is, however, rather to the traveller in the bays and fiords that we commend it—to one accustomed to the sea, and enjoying the sport which so much abounds in Norway. The invalid land traveller meets with many difficulties which are not encountered in boating besides those which are more or less common to both, viz., that of procuring a daily supply of fresh meat and other proper food. The only mode by which Norway may be advantageously visited by the class of persons under consideration is by yachting, and the period when it may be the most advantageously effected is from the beginning of June to the beginning of August.

SWITZERLAND AND THE TYROL.

The object which influences the visitors to Switzerland in the summer season is seldom that of health primarily, neither has it been common to direct thither the class of cases now under consideration, or, indeed, any class, for the precise object which we have in view. The variety of its scenery, the grandeur of its mountains, the beauty of its valleys, and the magnificence of its lakes, together with the manners of its inhabitants, must be the chief attractions. There are also, for many, a simple dietary and an increased amount of physical exertion, and for all a degree of lightness and purity of the atmosphere which is highly conducive to health; but the tendency of the whole is to lessen and not to increase the bulk of the body. The class of persons to be benefited in the ordinary mode of procedure are the sedentary and the full-fed, including those whose life is passed in the trouble and mental turmoil of a great town. But we are of opinion that, by a different plan, this may be used with advantage by those whose great desideratum is to increase the bulk of the body, and at the same time to increase in tone and vigour.

Every mountainous region may be divided, for the purpose of health, into two levels. In the lower there is much moisture, less movement of the air, greater atmospheric pressure upon the body, and the sensation of heat is greater. This level varies, in different localities, from an elevation of 1500 to 4000 feet, but commonly its higher limits may be stated at about 2500 feet. In the higher level the degree of moisture of the air is much reduced, and at the summits of the high mountains it is only in the degree observed in dry air. The pressure upon the body is less, the rate of pulsation and respiration is increased, as is probably, also, the depth of inspiration; the temperature is reduced, the hourly variations are greater, and the movement of the air is greater. The former condition is not suited to the class of patients under consideration, since the climate is mild and relaxing; but the latter is fitted for all such cases, except those in which there is much irritability of the air-passages or tendency to inflammation.

The whole of Switzerland is elevated much above the level of the sea, and, as we seek an elevated region, it might appear that all parts of it would be equally suitable, but this would be an error; for although even the lakes are situated at an elevation of much more than 1000 feet above the level of the sea, the temperature is there too great, at the summer season of the year, to admit of the advantages which we seek. It is therefore necessary to obtain a higher region still.

It is impossible for us to point out all the sites in Switzerland which are suitable for these cases; but, from the indications now offered, it will be understood that any position above 2500 feet will be proper, provided it be not too much exposed to cold wind, and offers the facilities for exercise and nutrition to which we have referred. We would, however, point out a few which, from our own knowledge, deserve attention; viz., Leukerbad, in the Rhone Valley; the Valley of Zermatt, near to the foot of Monte Rosa; the Valley of Unterwald, Lauterbrunnen; Kanderstag, at the foot of the Gemmi; Chamouni, Seelisberg, near Grüble, on the Rigi; the baths of Weissenberg, on the Simmerthal; and to these we may add many positions on the Jura Mountains.

We need not remark upon the advantage of choosing such situations as offer beauty and variety of scenery, and opportunities for attaining to yet higher elevations, since those conditions will be found almost universally; but it is important that the elevation should not approach to the limits of perpetual snow, and that it should be above the level of the lakes and streams.

11

The mode of life to be pursued is quite different to that followed by tourists, since it should be the aim to make only such an amount of exertion as is quite compatible with comfort, and almost with ease, and to take as large an amount as possible of the kind of food already recommended. In nearly all the Swiss villages there are opportunities of obtaining fresh meat, and in all, cows' and goats' milk, with cheese, ham, and honey are sufficiently abundant. There are, also, almost everywhere, opportunities of hiring mules or ponies for the purposes of exercise. Ample clothing should be at hand, and exposure to the midday sun avoided; and the aim should be to remain in one locality, and in a state of comparative rest. The period for such a visit is from the beginning of June to the end of August.

CHAPTER XLIII.

WINTER CLIMATES.

IN GREAT BRITAIN.

HERETOFORE, and particularly some years ago, the anxiety in reference to change of climate was limited to the selection of the winter residence. During the summer the cases were considered to do as well in any part of England as elsewhere, but in the winter it was desired to provide a milder atmosphere. This arose, no doubt, from the greater prevalence of inflammation than at present, and perhaps from attaching an undue importance to the cough ; but even now it is highly desirable that a winter residence in a comparatively mild climate should be obtained.

The period when the change from the summer to the winter climate should be made depends upon—1st, the condition of the case ; 2d, the character of the summer climate ; and, 3d, the distance of the proposed winter residence ; but the general rule to be adopted is to allow the cases in question to remain as long as possible in the summer climate. If there be much irritability of the air-passages, it will be necessary to seek a milder climate in September or the beginning of October. In ordinary cases, and in ordinary seasons, the patients may remain at Scarborough until November or December; at the Isle of Man until September or October; in Scotland until September; in Norway until August ; and in Switzerland until September or October, according to the elevation and latitude. But in all these instances the period of change should not be indicated by months, but by the state of the weather at the time and the healthful tolerance of the system.

When the winter residence is to be in England, and the patient is already here, the change may be made safely at any period of the year, from the rapidity of travelling and the protection from the weather; but if the patient be required to cross the Channel to come to England, or to go from England to the Continent, the change must be made not later than the middle of October. Hence, a winter residence in England enables those living in this country to remain at the summer and autumn residences for a longer period than when they are required to leave our shores; and, in accordance with the principles laid down, this must be considered as an advantage.

We will now point out a few of the most suitable places for winter residence, first in England, and then on the Continent of Europe.

VENTNOR.

We think that for the purpose in hand the first place must be given to Ventnor, both on account of its topographical and meteorological characters.

It is well known that Ventnor is placed on the sea coast, at a part of the Isle of Wight where there has been a very large land-slip, extending six miles in length, and offering sufficient width between the cliffs from which it has fallen and the sea for the purposes of residence and travelling. Hence, in front it is exposed to the open sea, with a south and southeasterly aspect, and is protected at the back by cliffs, some having a perpendicular face, and others rounded summits, 600 to 900 feet in height, from the north and northerly winds. It is not so low as the level of the sea, but has an elevation, varying up to nearly 150 feet. The soil consists chiefly of the alluvium and the detritus of lime and sandstone, and readily carries off the rain.

Hence, it offers a singular protection against the most injurious winds prevailing in the early part of the year; but it has the further very great advantage of enabling the resident to obtain a total change of atmosphere, when the weather will permit, by ascending the overhanging downs, and by travelling to the westerly side of the island. To this we attach the greatest importance, since the cases to which we refer only need shelter in a moderate degree; but they imperatively require the opportunity for active exertion, and for the acquisition of tone and vigour. We believe that no situation offers this combination of circumstances in a greater degree than Ventnor.

The following are the meteorological characters of Ventnor in the winter quarter, including January, February, and March, in the six years 1855 to 1860 inclusive, so carefully ascertained by Dr. Martin.

The average daily temperature was as follows :—

TABLE No. 21.

Mean Temperature.

	1855	1856	1857	1858	1859	1860
	°	°	°	°	°	°
January	38.7	42.6	40.	42.9	43.5	43.8
February	33.7	43.9	43.1	40.6	45.8	38.8
March	41.1	43.1	44.7	44.1	47.7	43.6
Mean	37.8	43.2	42.6	42.5	45.7	42.

Thus, in the average of six years the temperature of the quarter was 42 3°, whilst that at Greenwich was 38.8°.

The extremes of temperature during each month of the quarter were as follows :—

TABLE No. 22.

Extremes of Temperature.

		1855	1856	1857	1858	1859	1860
		°	°	°	°	°	°
January . .	Highest	53	52	53	53	52	53
	Lowest	25	29	25	26	31	30
February . .	Highest	49	54	55	53	55	51
	Lowest	21	30	29	29	34	26
March .	Highest	53	53	56	64	59	54
	Lowest	30	33	30	27	33	28

There was singular uniformity in the returns of the several years, and the extremes were 64° and 21°, yielding extremes of 43° in the course of six years.

The daily range of temperature is shown in the following table:—

TABLE No. 23.

Range of Temperature.

	1855	1856	1857	1858	1859	1860
	°	°	°	°	°	°
January	6.3	6.6	7.6	8.8	6.8	7.2
February	8.9	7.4	8.8	8.3	8.7	10.2
March	9.8	10.2	9.7	10.9	8.9	8.7
Mean	8.3	8.0	8.7	9.3	8.2	8.7

The daily range on the quarterly average was only 8.3°, as opposed to 12.1° at Greenwich.

The degree of saturation of the air by vapour was as follows, complete saturation being represented by 100°.

TABLE No. 24.

Saturation of the Air.

	1855	1856	1857	1858	1859	1860
January	84	86	77	82	86	81
February	83	90	86	81	82	77
March	81	76	84	80	78	80
Mean	83	84	82	81	82	79

The mean degree on the average of the quarter was 83°, and that at Greenwich was 85.2°.

The prevailing direction of the wind was E. and N.E., east variable in 1855, whilst the relative proportions of the winds in 1856 to 1860 were as follows :—

TABLE No. 25.

Prevalence of Winds.

	1856				1857				1858				1859				1860			
	N.	E.	S.	W	N.	E.	S.	W	N.	E.	S.	W	N.	E.	S.	W	N.	E.	S.	W
January . . .	7	9	...	12	9	5	3	11	6	7	8	10	4	6	5	16	3	7	7	14
February . . .	6	10	6	8	4	5	7	12	3	20	3	2	8	1	6	18	10	6	3	10
March . . .	4	28	2	1	4	8	5	14	5	11	3	12	5	1	6	19	6	2	8	15
Mean . . .	17	42	15	18	20	18	15	37	14	38	14	24	11	6	17	55	19	15	18	39

Thus it is shown that westerly and southwesterly winds were more prevalent than easterly and northeasterly in the proportion of 17 westerly to 12 easterly, and 25 southwesterly to 20 northeasterly. Hence it is evident that during the winter season easterly winds are frequent : but since the residents are protected by the cliffs and downs from all except the southeasterly, their frequency is not of great importance under ordinary circumstances.

Thus, on a review of the meteorological conditions of Ventnor, we find that the temperature is upwards of 40°, and, with one exception, higher than the most favoured parts of the kingdom. The daily range of temperature is small, but not so small as that at Scarborough or the Isle of Man (and, in some years, one or two other northern seaports), whilst the air is there drier than at almost any other place in the kingdom ; and, in addition to these facts, we must add its almost perfect shelter from the direct access of the cold winds. The only doubt which these conditions can raise in the mind is the effect of the dryness of the air, since in cases where there is any marked tendency to inflammatory action, that condition

would not be quite favourable. As it respects the vast majority of
the cases in question, there need, however, be no doubt as to the
fitness of the climate for them. Other parts of the Isle of Wight
partake to a considerable degree in the advantages of Ventnor, but
they lack the special protection which Ventnor claims. The general
temperature of the Isle of Wight at this season of the year is higher
than that of other parts of England, except Devonshire and Cornwall. Newport occupies an inland position, and Ryde is exposed to
easterly winds.

TORQUAY.

This beautiful sea-side sanatorium has certainly as great claims
to the designation of the Queen of Southern Watering-places as
Scarborough has to the Queendom of the North : and, in our judgment, no higher praise could be bestowed.

Torquay is situated upon the shores of a landlocked sheet of water
called Torbay, in the parallel of 50° 28′ N. latitude. It has a fine
sea-view, and offers excellent opportunities for boating on the bay
and for excursions upon the land, and abounds in interesting information for the geologist. The town itself is small, and situate
upon the shore, and in two ravines, which lead down to the level of
the sea. In the background, and on either hand, are high cliffs, of
which some present a bold and precipitous aspect to the sea, whilst
others have summits which, gradually rising in height, offer splendid
ranges of terraces, upon which have been built most commodious
villas. The lower town is occupied for the purposes of trade, whilst
in the beautiful panorama which extends itself on every side like
an extended fan above the town, are the residences for invalids and
for the wealthy inhabitants. The position is in the highest degree
picturesque, and it has had the good fortune to fall into the hands
of those who appreciate the beautiful, and who, with taste, talent, and
liberality, have turned its natural advantages to the best account.

The sea aspect is southwesterly, and as there are high cliffs on
every other side, the rising concavity in which the upper town is
built is protected from the north and east. The lower part of
the town is indeed so sheltered, that there is but little movement
in the air, except the wind be from the sea, and, consequently, in
hot weather the atmosphere is exceedingly oppressive ; but as we
ascend the beautifully-adorned terraces, we find a wider expanse
for the movement of the air, and, in the winter season, an expanded basin-like surface, courting the rays of the morning and
mid-day sun. The soil is warm and porous, and, from the rising
nature of the ground, there are great facilities for drainage. It is
also rich and highly cultivated.

The meteorological characters of Torquay are deserving of careful study, and manifest in a high degree its fitness for a winter
residence.

The average daily temperature in the three first months of the year in the years 1854 to 1860, excepting 1857 (the returns for 1857 having been omitted from the Registrar-General's Tables), was as follows :—

TABLE No. 26.

Mean Temperature.

	1854	1855	1856	1858	1859	1860
	°	°	°	°	°	°
January	42.9	38.8	43.3	42.8	45.8	43.1
February	42.6	38.5	44.7	41.4	45.7	38.6
March	45.3	40.2	42.5	43.4	47.4	43.6
Mean	43.6	37.5	43.5	42.5	46.3	41.7

The temperature in the year 1855 differed materially from that in the preceding and succeeding years; but upon the whole period we find that the temperature in the quarter was 42.5°. This was precisely the temperature recorded by us in reference to Ventnor.

The extremes of temperature during each month were as follows :—

TABLE No. 27.

Extremes of Temperature.

		1854	1855	1856	1858	1859	1860
		°	°	°	°	°	°
January .	Highest	54	52	52	53	52	53
	Lowest	29	28	29	25	33	31
February .	Highest	54	51	54	51	56	49
	Lowest	30	18	30	29	34	26
March .	Highest	57	52	53	59	58	58
	Lowest	34	30	33	27	34	28

The extremes of temperature during the quarter, on the average of five years, was 59° and 18°, giving an extreme of 40°.

The daily range of temperature was very small, as may be seen in the following figures :—

TABLE No. 28.

Daily Range of Temperature.

	1854	1855	1856	1858	1859	1860
	°	°	°	°	°	°
January	7.3	6.5	7.6	8.8	6.7	9.4
February	9.5	7.3	5.3	6.2	8.4	9.2
March	10.1	7.6	7.8	9.2	10.3	9.1
Mean	9.0	7.0	6.8	8.0	8.5	9.2

Thus, on the average of the three years, the mean daily range of temperature in the winter quarter was 8.1°, an amount scarcely less than that at Ventnor.

The degree of humidity compared with 100 representing saturation of the air was also low.

TABLE NO. 29.
Degree of Saturation of the Air.

	1854	1855	1856	1858	1859	1860
January	87	83	79	84	86	84
February	78	95	75	86	80	83
March	79	83	80	80	75	70
Mean	81	87	78	83	80	79

The average degree was 81, which was little less than that at
Ventnor.

Hence, on comparison of the meteorological characters of these
two principal southern Sanatoria, we are struck with their identity,
and arrive at the conclusion that either is well adapted for our purpose. Both, moreover, are places of singular beauty, and replete
with interest for the student of nature.

We do not purpose to continue an analysis of the characters of
the subordinate watering-places of the Devonshire coast, nor of
those of Truro and Penzance in Cornwall. They each, however,
possess all the general advantages of the climate, and differ chiefly
from Torquay in the absence of the particular kind of shelter from
the cold and easterly winds which that beautiful place possesses;
but, speaking generally, they offer many advantages to the class of
cases under consideration.

The mean temperature of the winter months in Devonshire and
Cornwall in the three years 1855, 1856, and 1857 was 41.4°, whilst
the mean daily range was 10.6°, and the mean degree of humidity
85°, conditions which must in this climate be regarded as very
favourable.

HASTINGS.

We now proceed to consider the advantages which attach to
Hastings as a winter residence for the cases of early phthisis. This
fashionable winter resort is divided into two parts by an artificial
line, the one comprehending the old town, and known as Hastings,
whilst the other has gradually extended itself along the shore until
it occupies an extent of two miles, and is known as St. Leonards.
Both lie very nearly on the level of the sea, and have a background
of cliffs, but the old town is built up to the foot of perpendicular
cliffs whilst the extension to St. Leonards has rounded cliffs, with
terraces arranged at various elevations. Hence the old town is
more strictly protected, and on the cliff offers the fine promenade of
the castle grounds; whilst the newer neighbourhood is more picturesque, has handsome buildings for the use of visitors, and possesses in front a fine sea promenade. It is therefore evident that

the advantages of the locality are offered in various degrees by the different parts of the town, and that a warmer and more sheltered or a cooler and more open position may be selected, according to the nature of the case and the will of the visitor. In reference to the class of cases under consideration, the St. Leonards neighbourhood is to be preferred; but on the occurrence of irritable cough or any evidence of inflammatory action, the old part of the town should be resorted to.

We turned to the Registrar-General's returns with a view to show the meteorological character of Hastings, but since 1856 there are no records from which we can make an analysis. The omission in the returns, and lately the absence of returns, is a most noticeable circumstance, and would lead the inquirer to form an unfavourable opinion of the locality.

THE CHANNEL ISLANDS.

There are four islands to which we might direct attention, viz., Jersey, Guernsey, Sark, and Alderney, each of which offers certain special advantages, but as only the two first are frequented by visitors, we shall restrict our remarks to them.

The islands are very small, and are situate rather off the French than the English coast, and as they lie in latitude 49° N., and are necessarily surrounded by water, we may expect to find them comparatively warm winter residences. They are well cultivated, and produce the most delicious fruits in the richest luxuriance. The native inhabitants are of French origin, and still retain French habits, so that visitors readily find pleasant society both amongst themselves and the residents.

We shall consider the meteorological characters of Jersey and Guernsey at the same time, since it will be found that either island is equally adapted for the class of cases now under consideration.

The average temperature of the air in the months of the winter quarter in these two islands was as follows; but owing to the absence of returns from Jersey for 1857, we have not been able to select the same years in reference to both places :—

TABLE No. 30.
Mean Temperature.

	Jersey.			Guernsey.		
	1854	1855	1856	1855	1856	1857
	°	°	°	°	°	°
January	42.2	39.	43.5	40.1	44.	42.5
February	42.5	35.2	43.7	36.5	43.5	41.7
March	44.8	40.6	41.7	51.4	41.2	43.3
Mean	43.2	38.3	42.9	39.3	42.9	42.5

The average temperature was thus the same in both islands, viz., 41.4° in Jersey, and 41.5° in Guernsey, and was nearly the same as that of Ventnor and Torquay.

The extremes of temperature during the same months were as follows :—

TABLE No. 31.

Extremes of Temperature.

		Jersey.			Guernsey.		
		1854	1855	1856	1855	1856	1857
		°	°	°	°	°	°
January . . .	Highest	51.	51.	52.	51.	51.5	52.
	Lowest	33.	28.	26.	27.	29.5	31.5
February . .	Highest	52.	49.	54.	49.	54.	49.5
	Lowest	30.	25.	31.	27.	32.	32.5
March	Highest	55.	52.	55.	53.	51.	54.
	Lowest	53.	30.	35.	33.5	36.5	34.

On looking at this table it is impossible not to notice the singular uniformity which occurs throughout the whole period, and the very small variation between the highest and lowest temperatures. There was no day in which the temperature in Jersey exceeded 55°, and in Guernsey 54°, whilst there was no day in which it fell lower than 25° in the former, and 27° in the latter. Hence the extreme range between the extremes of temperature during the winter months on the average of three years was only 30° in Jersey, and 27° in Guernsey—a condition much more favourable than occurs in the most sheltered parts of the shores of a larger country, as we have shown in reference to Ventnor and Torquay. This is no doubt due to the insular position and small size of the island, and the surrounding deep water.

The mean daily range of temperature in the two islands was as follows :—

TABLE No. 32.

Daily Range of Temperature.

	Jersey.			Guernsey.		
	1854	1855	1856	1855	1856	1857
	°	°	°	°	°	°
January	5.6	5.5	5 2	5.8	5.6	7.3
February	7 4	5 5	6.2	7.1	3.8	7.6
March	9.6	7.6	6.5	7.1	5.7	7 7
Mean	7.5	6.2	5.9	6.7	5.0	7.5

Uniformity of temperature is also well exemplified by this table, for on the average of the whole quarter the mean daily temperature varied only 6.5° and 6.4° in the two islands—a degree of uniformity which cannot be excelled.

It is well known that the influence of the wind is considerable on these islands, and that every wind must be a sea-wind to them. The direction is for the most part northeast or southwest, and during some part of the period of the year in question the prevailing direction is easterly, both in these islands and in England.

The degree of humidity is somewhat considerable, and is represented by the numbers constituting the following table, it being understood that full saturation of the air is represented by 100 :—

TABLE No. 33.
Degree of Saturation of the Air.

	Jersey.			Guernsey.		
	1854	1855	1856	1855	1856	1857
January	94	80	90	86	84	80
February	86	98	94	91	78	86
March	88	94	92	92	89	80
Mean	89	91	92	90	86	82

The average degree was thus ninety in Jersey, and eighty-six in Guernsey, and much exceeded that at Ventnor and Torquay.

On reviewing these meteorological characters, we perceive that the Channel Islands offer a warm and moist atmosphere, and are remarkable for the uniformity of their temperature. It must also be added that fogs prevail occasionally, as they must do when cool air is injected into a humid atmosphere. Hence it is a climate, when the easterly winds are absent, which is suited to those cases in which there is much irritability of the air passages, but for the ordinary class of cases it would be less tonic than the climate of Ventnor.

CLIFTON.

We purpose to refer only to another home winter climate, viz., that of Clifton, which in some respects offers a contrast with that just discussed. Clifton is situate upon the hills bordering the deep gorge of the Avon, leading to the Bristol Channel, and whilst fully exposed to the southeast wind is sheltered from the westerly gales of the Atlantic. The surface is very undulating, so that the lower part is sheltered, whilst the downs are very exposed, and hence some care is required in selecting the part of the locality suited to each case. It is wooded, and offers much variety of aspect, and is indeed one of the prettiest localities in the country. It offers every facility for surface drainage by its undulations, and also for subsoil drainage from the nature of the rock upon which it rests.

The meteorological characters are as follows in the winter months.

The average temperature of the air was lower than that hitherto recorded by us.

TABLE No. 34.

Mean Temperature.

	1855	1856	1857	1858	1859	1860
	°	°	°	°	°	°
January	36.2	40.	37.3	38 5	41.3	39.9
February	29.3	41.7	39.5	36.	42.9	36.1
March	37.9	39.6	41.8	41.2	45.5	40 8
Mean	34.5	37.1	39.4	38.6	43.2	38.9

The mean temperature during the three years was only 38.6°, which was not only much below that already recorded, but was a little less than that at Greenwich.

The extremes of temperature were considerable.

TABLE No. 35.

Extremes of Temperature.

		1855	1856	1857	1858	1859	1860
		°	°	°	°	°	°
January . . .	Highest	51.4	52 5	51.3	53.8	55.	56.
	Lowest	22.2	21.9	16.7	21.	26.5	26.2
February .	Highest	48.4	55.5	51.8	51.	55.	48.9
	Lowest	11.5	23.8	20.3	21.	28.6	23.1
March .	Highest	55.3	57.1	50 1	66.3	58.8	53.9
	Lowest	23.1	24.4	25.3	20.9	27.3	21.7

The highest temperature was 66.3° and the lowest 11.5°, so that the range of the extremes during the period was 55.5°.

The mean daily range of temperature was moderate, viz., 10.5°, as shown in the following table.

TABLE No. 36.

Daily Range of Temperature.

	1855	1856	1857	1858	1859	1860
	°	°	°	°	°	°
January	6.5	8.1	8.5	10.4	8.5	9.5
February	10.1	9.6	11.7	9.6	11.3	11.4
March	12.4	13 5	12 9	14.9	10.2	12.1
Mean	9.7	10.	11.	11.6	10.	11.

The degree of humidity was not considerable, and corresponds closely with that observed at Greenwich, viz., 86° at the former and 85.2° at the latter, but it was greater than that recorded at Ventnor and Torquay.

TABLE No. 37.

Degree of Saturation of the Air.

	1855	1856	1857	1858	1859	1860
January	93	90	89	86	92	91
February	80	92	90	84	85	79
March	88	82	85	82	87	90
Mean	90	88	88	84	88	86

Thus the climate of Clifton in the winter months is less warm and of far greater vicissitude than that of Ventnor, Devonshire, and the Channel Islands. It is drier than the latter, and less dry than the two former. Hence its character is rather tonic and stimulating, and not suited to those early cases of phthisis where there is much irritability of the air passages. There are certain cases of that disease for which it is fitted; but all such persons should occupy sheltered houses, and expose themselves to the air of the downs on fine and warm days.

REVIEW OF BRITISH CLIMATES.

On a review of the characters of the climates to which we have referred, we consider that Ventnor and Torquay occupy the first places in reference to the mass of persons afflicted with early phthisis. The more robust may winter at Clifton, and the more sensitive may select the Channel Islands.

FOREIGN CLIMATES.

In selecting a foreign winter and early spring residence for the class of patients under consideration, we must seek for the conditions which will enable the patient to spend his time in the open air, and such are chiefly the temperature, dryness of the air, and the violence of the winds. Speaking generally, those climates will be the most suitable in which the air is not moist, the temperature never very high nor low, but uniformly sustained, and where the easterly winds do not greatly prevail. In all these respects there is much diversity in the climates which we shall proceed to notice; and we shall much more frequently find that a particular locality offers both prejudicial and beneficial characters, rather than the precise conditions which we need. It is not necessary for our purpose to enter at length into the characters of foreign climates, nor

to refer to a large number of localities, but we shall content ourselves with specifying those places which seem to us to be the best
fitted, and with indicating their leading characters.

THE NILE.

We are, upon the whole, disposed to place the Nile in the first
rank of suitable climates, on account of the elevation of its temperature and the dryness and elasticity of the air in its upper
part.

The period of the year to proceed from this country to the Nile
is the middle or end of October, and the best mode is by the Penin-
sular and Oriental Company's steamers, although some prefer to
travel through Spain on the way. The voyage to Alexandria is
made in about a month. It is then usual to proceed at once to
Cairo, and engage a dragoman and a boat for the journey up the
Nile; or, if it is very early, to select a boat at Alexandria, and
proceed on to Cairo. As it is desirable that the invalid should have
as little trouble as possible, it will be the most convenient to pay
the dragoman a stipulated sum per day, on condition that he
secures the boat which the traveller prefers, and engages the first
and second captains and sailors, and supplies daily provisions according to a written scale. The journey from Cairo should commence from the middle of November to the beginning of December;
and as it is usual for two or more persons to join in the expense of
the boat, it will avoid delay if the party could be made up before
reaching Cairo. The journey should be made with a moderate degree of rapidity until the traveller arrive at Thebes, and in Nubia
he will find the atmosphere in its driest and most elastic state. In
this part of the journey he will do well to linger, and proceed leisurely to the second cataract. The return journey should not commence before the middle or end of February, so as to terminate at
Cairo at the end of March.

The general character of the climate during the journey will be
found to correspond with an ordinary summer in England, with the
sun's rays somewhat hotter and the nights cooler than in this northern climate. The disadvantages, in reference to the climate, are
the hot sun and the cool nights causing a considerable range of
temperature; and if the return journey be made early, cold winds
will be met with below Thebes. Hence it is necessary that there be
a sufficiency of warm clothing. The journey is also manifestly
more fitted for gentlemen than ladies, since the former may amuse
themselves by sporting, or by wandering along the banks of the Nile,
whilst the sailors drag the boat along; but the latter are necessarily
more restricted to the boat. There is not much difficulty in obtaining good provisions: but the milk, being obtained from the buffalo,
has a rich and peculiar flavour, and does not agree, unless it be first
skimmed, with certain states of dyspepsia. Whilst, therefore, ex-

treme dyspeptics, or persons much enfeebled or liable to diarrhœa, should not undertake this journey, we think that the mass of persons afflicted with early phthisis will be benefited by it.

As the termination of the return journey occurs so early as the beginning of April, it is necessary that the patient proceed to Italy before he returns to England.

PAU.

Pau is a city containing upwards of twenty thousand inhabitants, situate in the Pyrenees, at an elevation of 150 feet above the river Gave. It is about twenty miles distant from the mountains, and 125 miles south of Bordeaux. It is now within a forty-eight hours' journey of England, and may be reached by railway, except the last few miles, for which diligences are provided from the Aire Station, to carry the passengers through in four hours. On approaching the city from the north side, the mountains may be seen extending over a distance of sixty miles, and as to the general beauty of the locality we may follow Dr. Taylor's excellent example, and cite the opinion of Mr. Inglis. He says: "It has always enjoyed the reputation of being one of the most interesting cities of the south of France, and altogether I think it deserves its reputation. It lies in one of the most beautiful and most abundant countries of Europe, in one of the first climates; and the city itself is clean, airy, and abounds in every convenience, and in most luxuries. As for the environs of Pau, they are certainly beautiful. The Gave serpentines through the charming undulating country that surrounds the town; grain, meadows, and vines diversify the scenery, and innumerable country houses are everywhere scattered around. Nothing can exceed the beauty of the promenades in the neighbourhood of Pau. Some lie along the edge of the Gave, others along the banks of the smaller river, and within the town there is a large and shaded platform which commands a magnificent view over the surrounding country."

The climate of Pau is somewhat cold in the early winter months; but in the later ones and the early spring, it is warm, dry, and fine, and corresponds with our Devonshire climate. The city is protected from the north by the gradual ascent of the Landes of the Pont Long, and is not very liable to oppressive southerly winds. It is remarkably free from any violence of wind, since the neighbouring mountain peaks divide the current, and direct it at an elevation far above the town. The air is clear, and whilst changes of weather are frequent, they are evanescent also. The degree of humidity at the season of the year under consideration is considerable, varying as the east or north wind blows, but it does not produce fog.

It appears from Dr. Ottley's observations during eight years, as quoted by Dr. Taylor, that the meteorological characters of Pau are very favourable.

The *mean temperature* in the autumn and winter months was as follows :—

Oct.	Nov.	Dec.	Jan.	Feb.	Mar.
56.5°	46.9°	42.5°	40.5°	43.2°	47.9°

which affords an average temperature of 48.6° and 43.8° in the two quarters.

The difference between *means of the extremes of temperature was*—

Oct.	Nov.	Dec.	Jan.	Feb.	Mar.
15.3°	13.4°	11.°	12.°	13.5°	14.8°

The *degree of humidity of the air* was as follows, saturation being represented by 100 :—

Oct.	Nov.	Dec.	Jan.	Feb.	Mar.
80	81	83	82	81	79

'The general characters of the climate are those of softness and mildness, allaying nervous and vascular excitability, which, within moderate limits, are such as the cases of early phthisis need in the winter season, but its tendency is to produce a certain degree of relaxation, and therefore the residence should not be prolonged to a later period than April or May. The period to arrive at Pau is the end of October or the middle of November.

In reference to the cases of early phthisis to which the climate of Pau is suited, we scarcely see grounds to make any selection, for there is perhaps no place which offers a better climate in the early spring, and although during the winter the temperature is below that of Devonshire, it is perhaps sufficiently warm. If the patient be moderately robust, he may more freely expose himself to the cooler temperature of December and January, and may indeed, if he be fond of sport, follow the hounds ; whilst those who are less robust, or who suffer more from irritability of the air-passages, should arrive at Pau later, or, being there, should limit their period of exercise to the middle hours of the day. It is not a climate in which tone is gained, but it is one in which loss of tone and health in the winter may be avoided.

MADEIRA.

The characters of the climate of Madeira are so well known that it is not necessary to enter into any detail, but we may state that generally it is remarkable for mildness and uniformity of temperature, with a considerable degree of humidity of the air (as determined by its approach to saturation), clearness, and absence of fogs. In November and December the climate is clear, dry, and fine, and until February it is nearly all that can be desired, but in the spring there is great liability to easterly winds, and the climate is then in its least valuable state.

The different degrees of elevation of the island enable the resident to live in almost any climate, since by ascending he finds a higher temperature, and hence this island is one of the very few places in which a patient may remain for a lengthened period. We have not included it in our list of summer climates, but a patient residing there during the winter may remain during the summer also, if he can escape the evil influence of the spring season. The range of temperature throughout the year is unusually small.

ALGERIA.

Whilst Madeira has perhaps lost somewhat of public favour during the last fifteen years, as other places of resort have urged their claims, Algeria has been brought into notice as a winter residence for cases of early phthisis, and seems likely to attract numerous patients. The French government have authorized a long series of inquiries to be made as to the nature of the climate, and the results speak favourably of it for persons afflicted with chest diseases. We do not purpose to enter upon the discussion of the whole country, since the information upon it is as yet very meagre. The country is very extensive, and portions of it not very secure, but we shall extract the meteorological character of Algiers from the interesting work recently issued by Dr. Scoresby Jackson, of Edinburgh. (Table No. 38.)

Hence it appears that we have in Algiers a climate of high average winter temperature, of a moderate degree of daily range of temperature, and of high and steady barometric indications. The prevailing direction of the wind is westerly in the months under consideration, but northerly winds are common, and the north-westerly wind is a modified *mistral*. The southwesterly wind is rainy, and there is a large rainfall, but chiefly in sleet and heavy showers.

TABLE No. 38.
Meteorology of Algiers.

	Autumn.			Winter.		
	Oct.	Nov.	Dec.	Jan.	Feb.	Mar.
	°	°	°	°	°	°
Mean temperature . . .	73.85	66.40	60.82	59.18	59.01	60.05
Mean daily range	15.84	10.08	12.06	13.86	12.06	10.08
Barometer (inches) . . .	30.095	30.005	30.088	30.045	30.039	30.018

	Quarter.	
	Autumn.	Winter.
	°	°
Mean temperature	67.09	59.41
Mean daily range	12.69	12.0
Barometer (inches)	30.061	30.034

NICE AND NAPLES.

We have classed these two beautiful sea-side resorts together because there is some similarity in their climates, and they are only fitted for a limited class of cases.

The temperature is sufficiently high, viz., 48° at Nice during the winter months, but in the spring season cold and easterly winds prevail in both places. The range of temperature of the day is very small at Nice, and not considerable at Naples. The degree of saturation of the air is moderate in Nice, and more considerable at Naples, but the character of the climate is rather that of dryness. Nice is so surrounded by mountains that it is much sheltered from westerly and easterly winds, and from the *mistral*, whilst Naples suffers from the sirocco. Hence the conditions of the mid-winter months are not unfavourable, but from the end of February they are not such as are well suited to cases of phthisis.

The class of cases which may winter there are those in whom there is no predisposition to inflammatory action, and to whom occasional cold winds are not injurious, and whilst the occurrence of inflammation is not a leading character in cases of early phthisis, it is a circumstance so much to be avoided that only a few cases could with propriety spend the later winter and early spring months there.

MENTONE.

This little village, situated within a few miles of Nice, has been known for some years as a locality far better suited than Nice as a winter residence for persons affected with diseases of the chest, from the great shelter which it affords; but it is only during the last two or three years that professional attention has been widely directed to it. The experience of Dr. H. Bennett, and the favourable opinion which Dr. De Pascali has formed of it, have induced many to avail themselves of the advantages; and whilst some will doubtless go there to whom it is not suited, it is probable that the class of cases now under consideration, in whom there is no marked inflammatory tendency, may find it beneficial. The immediate neighbourhood and the line of sea coast, are interesting, and offer convenience for drives and promenades, and suitable accommodation is now prepared for a limited number to pass the winter with comfort.

The leading character of the climate at the season under consideration is that of mildness, which includes a tolerably high temperature with a somewhat considerable approach to saturation of the air. It is warm without being relaxing, and there is no prevalence of fog. Dr. Bennett states, in his work on Mentone, that the town is sheltered from the north and northerly winds, but southerly winds are often violent. The sun is hot, and the nights are cool. There is neither frost nor fog. The sky is clear, and there are but few rainy days. Yet, whilst the days are commonly warm and dry, there are sometimes drizzling days, in which the weather resembles that of a November day in England. Dr. Edwin Lee, in a recent work, has pointed out the advantages and disadvantages of Mentone, and has shown that in the summer it is relaxing, and in the winter stimulating.

ROME.

This ancient city, with its unequalled monuments of art, offers a very good inland winter residence, since its winter and spring temperature is sufficiently elevated, and the uniformity of temperature is very striking. The degree of saturation of the air is considerable, so that its character in the months in question is soft to a considerable degree. There is no prevalence of wind from any quarter, but occasionally there are sufficiently high, dry, and cold northerly winds.

Hence the class of cases to which it is well suited are those who suffer from irritability of the air-passages, who have much general sensibility of system, and who have taste to appreciate and study the *chef-d'œuvres* of ancient art. The principal objection to Rome for persons of only moderate means, is the necessity for leaving England early, so as to make the long journey by easy stages; but if this can be readily effected, the journey will offer the enjoyment of the climate of southern France and the Mediterranean before the patient reach his winter residence.

CHAPTER XLIV.

It may seem to be superfluous to introduce a chapter upon prognosis in a work which professes to treat of a curable disease, but as there are many questions upon which the wished-for issue depends besides the stage of the disease, we think it will be convenient to discuss this subject separately.

The conditions in which we may confidently hope for a successful result are the following, when they are all present at the same time :—

1. The disease in the stage preceding any evidence of the deposition of tubercle, or when the amount of tubercle deposited is very small and isolated at the apex of one lung.
2. The progress of the disease has been slow, so that there have been evidences of slight failure of the general system during many months, and with no evidence of a recently accelerated rate.
3. The original state of the constitution was moderately good.
4. The age from about twenty years to middle life.
5. The existing state of the health still moderately good, so that, by careful regulation, a due amount of nitrogenous food and of exertion may be taken with comfort.
6. The rate of pulsation and respiration not materially varied from that of health.
7. Cheerful willingness to obey the prescribed directions, and such a pecuniary and domestic position that the whole arrangements necessary to the treatment of the case may be carried out.
8. Due freedom from anxiety, and removal from whatever conditions are unfavourable to the restoration to health.

Such are the most favourable conditions, and it must further be observed that they are met with in a large proportion of cases in

the middle and upper classes of society, but they cannot be universal. We will now enumerate the several circumstances which are
unfavourable, and the degree of importance which should be attached
to them.

THE LUNGS.

*When the deposit is increased so that it may be detected below the
clavicle.*

The extent of the deposit is important, both from the interference
with the vital functions of the lungs, and from affording grounds for
the occurrence of new complications; but under these conditions
there is ground for hope if the amount of deposit does not appear
to be great, so as to interfere much with the circulation of the blood
in the parts thus occupied, if the progress have been slow and
uniform, and all other conditions are favourable. We attach far
greater importance to the aggregation of a solid mass of tubercle in
a moderate space than to an equal quantity distributed in small
masses, and yet not spread over a large area.

When the deposit is met with in both apices.

We think that it cannot admit of a doubt that the progress of the
case is greater, and the prognosis more unfavourable, when there is
a small amount of deposit in both lungs, than when only one lung
is implicated in the same, or even in a somewhat greater degree.
This would probably imply that the causes of the disease exerted
a more general influence, or were more intense, as we should certainly infer that there was double danger of complications. Yet
when the deposit is very small, and all other conditions satisfactory,
the case is still hopeful.

When softening has already occurred.

We have limited the curable conditions to those in which the extent of softening is small, and yet involving the whole tubercle then
deposited. We have seen cases in which these conditions existed,
and every mark of disease has passed away except a certain degree
of unevenness of the vesicular murmur over the part. We have,
however, the conviction that softening in any degree very seriously
complicates the case, and it is then only under most favourable circumstances that we can hope for the removal of the softened matter,
whether with or without the production of a cavity, which may remain open for a period. In such cases it is impossible to give a
favourable prognosis except by watching the progress of the case,
but when it is found that the softening is strictly limited, that the evidences of it gradually pass away, that the vesicular murmur is gradually restored by the increased degree of expansion of the surrounding
cells, and that no further deposition of tubercle occurs, a favourable
issue may be anticipated.

*When the feebleness of respiration is very great, so that there is
general flattening of the chest.*

It not unfrequently occurs that the degree of diminution of respi-

12

ratory power and action is very great, without there being any evidences of tubercular deposition, and in such instances there is marked prostration of the whole nervous system. This is much more common in females than in males, but in both it is particularly found in those who pursue strictly sedentary occupations, attended by much anxiety and poor living, as, for example, sempstresses, tailors, and shoemakers.

When the patient cannot fully pursue the system of deep inspiration, whether from want of respiratory power or of appreciation as to the right method of performing it.

We have already intimated that many such cases are met with in which, with all the training which can be given, the respiratory action is short, quick, and gasping, when an attempt is made to adopt the plan of deep respiration. It is difficult to dissociate these two conditions; but we have no doubt that in many persons who have pursued sedentary occupations sedulously for years, and who have lost much courage and nervous power, they have lost the method of easy and deep respiration—in other words, have forgotten how to breathe. In such instances, the chest falls in expiration below the normal degree, so that there is a less amount of residual air remaining in the lungs, and hence the diminution in the vital processes, and the difficulty of maintaining a due degree of expansion of the lung, are proportionally increased. Unless such patients can be taught to inspire slowly and deeply, so as to expand the air cells, and also to keep them expanded from that time, at the end of inspiration we believe the case to be hopeless.

When hæmoptysis is persistent without any evidence of progress of the disease, or when the disease progresses very slowly.

We have had numerous cases under our constant care for two or three years in which the disease appeared to be kept in abeyance, and the general health improved, but in which there was, from time to time, attacks of hæmoptysis, and ultimately the signs of progress appeared. The importance of this indication is no doubt in reference to the want of freedom of circulation in the lungs as a whole, which attends deficient expansion, or the state of the blood and general organism, whereby a healthy condition of nutrition is not regained. It occurs without any sign whatever of softening of any tubercle which may have been deposited.

THE GENERAL SYSTEM.

When the powers of the general system are greatly enfeebled.

When the capability of reaction is found by experience to be very small.

When the appetite, digestion, or assimilation is very defective, and particularly when milk, fat, and other kinds of animal food, cannot be sufficiently taken even after careful training.

When food, clothing, or shelter is deficient in any marked degree.

When there is oppressing anxiety.

When the patient cannot be removed from injurious conditions, such as foul or heated air, exposure to cold, and sedentary occupations.

When self-abuse in either sex is, or has been, largely practised, or alcoholic liquors or smoking largely indulged in.

When the system is highly sensitive, so that the whole organization is in a state of perpetual unrest, or when it is so deficient in nervous sensibility and activity that it does not respond readily to the ordinary stimuli.

When the patient is younger or older than that indicated.

When from any cause the patient will not or cannot obtain change of climate, and will not or cannot steadily pursue the prescribed plan of treatment.

We have not thought it necessary to offer separate comments under these heads, since the whole form a connected series, and any of them is sufficient to greatly lessen, or perhaps extinguish, hope in the prognosis of the case. We attach so much importance to these several questions, that we advise the most careful consideration of each one of them, and as the opinion to be formed respecting them is one of degree, it is often necessary that the case be watched for a time before a correct judgment can be formed.

The importance of age seems to be less theoretically than practically. In persons aged twelve to fifteen years, or thereabouts, in whom the evidences of phthisis exist, we have found the disease less capable of arrest or cure than in those at a later age. This may be owing to the fact that the early attack of the disease may be in some degree evidence of the deep implication of the system, and probably it may be in part due to complications which arise in reference to the appearance of the menses, and the various rapid changes which occur in the organism and the passions at the period of puberty. But however it may be explained we augur less favourably of a case in which the disease begins before æt. 16, than of one in whom it is deferred until twenty years of age or later. The unfavourable prognosis in advanced age is clearly associated with the progressing defect of the vital powers, the diminution in the expansibility of the lung which always proceeds at that period, and the diminished possibility of adopting some of the means which are necessary to a cure.

There is an important relation between the state of the lungs and the general system, which we must always consider when forming a prognosis. A small amount of lung disease, with a very enfeebled system, is far more unfavourable than a somewhat larger amount of the former, with a moderately robust state of the latter. Whilst there are many cases in which the general health appears to be moderately good when the lung disease is far advanced, the general rule is to find the system injured whilst the lung disease is yet very limited, and hence, after having ascertained that the latter is restricted within the narrow limits already indicated as hopeful, the whole question of prognosis rests upon the state of the general system.

CHAPTER XLV.

GENERAL AND NUMERICAL CONDITIONS.

WE purpose under this head to introduce a short summary of facts derived from a very extensive inquiry into the conditions which may be presumed to have modified the constitution of phthisical persons *when in health*, and to which reference has already been made in several parts of this work. The primary aspect of this inquiry is that of etiology, and had it been our purpose to have entered specially upon the causation of phthisis, we should doubtless have referred to the inquiry under that head, but as it has an important bearing upon prognosis in reference to the constitution of the patients, we purpose to insert the results in this place. We do not, however, intend to enter into much detail, since the computations were made only when this work was half through the press, and the subject has been treated at due length in a paper read before the Royal Medical and Chirurgical Society on March 20, 1826.

The inquiry embraced 1000 patients, of whom 600 were males and 400 females, and extended over several years. It was altogether made by ourself, and the diagnosis of phthisis in a marked stage of consolidation or of destruction was made by our colleagues or ourself. We will first consider the circumstances which refer to the parents, and then those belonging to the patients.

Fifty-four per cent. had lost the father, 46 per cent. the mother, and 28 per cent. had lost both parents. In 25 per cent. only were both parents living. Their average age at death was 50.8 years, with an increased duration of 4.7 years on the part of the fathers. The most frequent age at death was 35 to 55 years, whilst only 11 per cent. died under æt. 35, and some lived to upwards of æt. 95. 18 per cent. had experienced feeble health before the birth of the patient, and 34 per cent. throughout life. In 22 7 per cent. one or both parents had led unsteady lives, 21.1 per cent. of the parents had died of consumption, whilst in 2.8 per cent. the grand parents, in 23.3 per cent. the brothers or sisters, and in 9.1 per cent. the uncles or aunts had died of the same disease. They had suffered from rheumatism in 22 per cent., from asthma in 9.4 per cent., from liver disease and gout in 9. and 7.2 per cent., and from fevers, ague, insanity, and diabetes in between 4 and 5 per cent. Presumed scrofulous affections were extremely rare. In only six cases was there consanguinity of the parents.

The age of the parents at the birth of the patient was, in half of the cases, from æt. 25 to æt. 35, and only in 2 per cent. was it less than æt. 20. The number of children was very large, viz., an average of 7.5 to a family, and in some families there were 23 children. The patient was the first child in twenty per cent., and the first, second, or third child in half of the whole cases. 40 per cent. of the parents' children had died.

Hence, in reference to questions involved in the idea of hereditary predisposition, it has been proved that in a large proportion of the cases the parents died in the middle of life, and had had feeble health. Their children had died in large proportion, and consumption occurred in one-fifth of the parents. But in all these matters there was a large proportion in which there was no evidence of feeble health or direct tendency to phthisis. The parents did not marry too early or too late, and the patient was neither the result of immaturity nor of senile exhaustion, so far as age may indicate those conditions, yet he was commonly amongst the earliest children born to them. They were unusually prolific.

The question of hereditary taint implies either the direct transmission of the elements of phthisis to the child, or a state of system in which phthisis is pre-eminently liable to occur. Neither of these ideas are supported by the results now given, as applicable to this class of cases as a whole, for they support the previously recorded statements of Dr. Walshe, that the hereditary transmission of phthisis from the parents, in hospital patients, is much less frequent than had previously been asserted. The results show that no one condition is dominant, but that phthisical patients are a mixed class of the community.

The average age of the patients at the period of the inquiry was 28.8 years, and 44 per cent. of the whole were between twenty and thirty years of age. In only 13 per cent. were they under æt. 20, and a few were æt. 60. 24 per cent. had been feeble at birth, but only 22 per cent. had suffered from feebleness of the general health, and 17 per cent. from generally defective appetite. In 12.6 per cent. the lungs had always been delicate. Only 2.5 per cent. had been dry nursed, 25.4 per cent. had perspired very freely, and 25 had never worn flannel next the skin. 16, 65.4, 60, and 41 per cent. had not had measles, scarlet fever, smallpox, and hooping-cough in their order, and the frequency of any long-continued ill effects from these diseases was insignificant. 12.8 per cent. had suffered from enlarged glands, and 4.5 per cent. from affections of the eyes, but otherwise the evidences of scrofulous diseases scarcely existed. 16.7 per cent. had suffered from inflammation of the lungs, and 14.8 per cent. from rheumatism, whilst typhus fever and frequent diarrhœa had occurred in 8.0 per cent., ague in 5.6 per cent., and liver disease in 4.3 per cent. of the cases.

43.5 per cent were married, and of these 13 per cent. were up to the period of the inquiry childless. Their average age at the birth

of their first child was from æt. 20 to æt. 25, and in only 9 per cent.
were they under æt. 20.   The number of children was one and two
in 44 per cent. and one, two, and three in 55 per cent.   38 per cent.
of the children had died, and in 43 per cent. the general state of the
health of the children was bad.   Abortion had occurred in 46.2 per
cent. of the child-bearing married women, and some had suffered
eight abortions.

11.6 per cent. had committed sexual abuse, 18.2 per cent. had
masturbated, and 22 per cent. had suffered from involuntary emissions.   16 per cent. had had syphilis, and 38.5 per cent. gonorrhœa.   29.6 per cent. had led a bad life at some period, 24.5 per cent.
had drank to excess, and 48 per cent. had smoked tobacco. 19.3 per
cent. had submitted to late hours, and 22.2 per cent. had suffered
much anxiety.   In 70 per cent. there was some complaint as to the
injurious influence of their occupations, and of those causes exposure
long hours, close and hot rooms, bending posture, and dust or fumes
were complained of in 32.1, 28.6, 24.4, 20 and 15.8 per cent. in
their order.   9 per cent. had taken mercury largely, and 54.4
per cent. had been bled at the arm from one to twelve times.

Thus, a large proportion of the patients had been born feeble, had
had feeble and short-lived children, had suffered from the effects of
injurious occupations, and had been injured by the anxieties and
immoralities of life.   They were thus influenced by original and
acquired causes of disease; but however important the former might
be, it is impossible not to admit that the latter was still more so.
They had not suffered from early marriages, and considering their
average age, they had been sufficiently prolific, although no incon-
siderable proportion had been sterile.

Hence, again, we cannot but regard phthisical patients as a very
mixed class of persons, and one which derives its causes of disease
from a great variety of diverse conditions, many of which are, however, within their control and preventible.   The proportion of those
who had suffered from general feeble health and insufficient appetite
throughout life was very small, but as they were the judges it may
be that their standard of health was low.

One striking feature to which we must refer was the greater liability of the female over the male sex to many of the ills to which
we have referred.   Thus, in reference to the parents, more mothers
than fathers had children early, had feeble general health, and had
died early.   Of the patients, more females than males had mothers
who died early, had most relatives who had died of phthisis, had
parents with one child only, had experienced feeble health and defective appetite through life, had had delicacy of the lungs, were married when very young, had feeble children, had lost most children,
had suffered from anxiety, had had measles, scarlet fever, and hooping-cough, had not worn flannel next the skin, had a very defective
education, were of susceptible temperament, had brown eyes, florid
complexion, and fleshy habit, and had suffered from coldness of the

extremities.   This is most striking evidence of the liability of females to conditions tending to constitutional disease.

We may now ask, in conclusion, in what way may we regard these inquiries as important in reference to prognosis?   It may be fairly replied that, whatever will so affect the constitution as to induce a disease, will, when the disease exists, be so many reasons against the cure; and hence, in estimating the probability of cure of any disease, it is requisite to weigh well the relative importance of the causes which may have induced it.   The first requisite in forming a prognosis in the early or curable stage of phthisis, is to ascertain the leading conditions to which the disease may have been due, with a view to ascertain the degree of their influence over the constitution, and the probability of their removal ; and hence, instead of regarding the cases as belonging to one class of persons, it will be found that they are exceedingly multiform and varied.   The first place must doubtless be given to such as originally affected the system, and to the sex, so that of those patients whose parents and relatives have exhibited special marks of disease or of defective constitutions, whether phthisical or otherwise, and females, the prognosis must be less favourable.   So also we must give a first rank to a defective state of the system of the patient commencing in early life and long continuing, from whatever cause it might have arisen. The importance of the acquired causes of disease must be estimated by their intensity and continuance, as well as by the natural vigour of the constitution and the effect which they have produced upon it. As a whole, their position must be secondary to that of those just referred to ; but those which acted before adult life, and which then injured the health—as sexual excess and masturbation—are of prime importance.   We are, therefore, of opinion that in every case there should be careful inquiry into the circumstances now referred to, and that the probability of cure will rest as much upon it as upon the more minute examination of the lungs, and the impression as to the state of the general system of the patient.

INDEX.